The Patient Was Vietcong

The Patient Was Vietcong

An American Doctor in the Vietnamese Health Service, 1966–1967

LAWRENCE H. CLIMO, M.D.

McFarland & Company, Inc., Publishers

Jefferson, North Carolina

LIBRARY OF CONGRESS CATALOGUING-IN-PUBLICATION DATA

Climo, Lawrence H.
    The patient was Vietcong : an American doctor in the Vietnamese
Health Service, 1966–1967 / Lawrence H. Climo, M.D.
        p.   cm.
    Includes bibliographical references and index.

    ISBN 978-0-7864-7899-6
    softcover : alkaline paper ∞

    1. Climo, Lawrence H.   2. Vietnam War, 1961–1975—
Medical care.   3. Vietnam War, 1961–1975—Personal narratives,
American.   4. United States. Army—Medical personnel—
Biography.   5. Physicians—United States—Biography.
6. Humanitarian assistance—Vietnam—History—20th century.
7. United States. Military Assistance Command, Vietnam.
Military Provincial Health Assistance Program.   I. Title.

    DS559.44.C55 2014
    959.704'37092—dc23
    [B]   2013044219

BRITISH LIBRARY CATALOGUING DATA ARE AVAILABLE

Front cover: the outpatient entrance to the civilian section
of Dar Lac province hospital; *inset* the author outside the outpatient
clinic; with dates: the Military Assistance Command, Vietnam
(MACV) badge

Manufactured in the United States of America

*McFarland & Company, Inc., Publishers
   Box 611, Jefferson, North Carolina 28640
      www.mcfarlandpub.com*

Table of Contents

Acknowledgments

The details in this book, which covers my two years of military service from 1965 to 1967, were drawn from the frequent and lengthy journal/letters I sent home during those years. My parents, Doctor Samuel Climo and Esther Levitin Climo, my younger sister, Doctor Ann Climo Fernbach, and my older brother and sister-in-law, Doctor Merrill Climo and Barbara Heifetz Climo, saved my letters over the years. When each, in turn, reached retirement age and began down-sizing, they returned my letters to me. My girlfriend, then fiancée (and, upon my return, my bride), Diane Schwartz Climo, likewise saved all my letters. This account would not have been possible without the recovery of those detailed letters.

Additional contributions included personal communications from William Baxley, Michael Benge, Hank Brown, John Guingrich, Donald Horsburgh, Daniel Melberg, Ngyyen Dang Hoan, Nguyen Ngoc Chinh, Alfonso Rodriguez, Lehman Strickland, Ton That Niem, and Katherine Vo.

Thanks to the *Berkshire Eagle*, which gave permission to reproduce in full the feature articles that tell an important part of this story.

Introduction

Some years ago I was invited to a party of friends. We were all nearing retirement age and, to make the party interesting as well as fun, were asked to wear to the party what we wore in the 1960s. The Vietnam War was the seminal event of that decade and our young adult lives; we came to that party wearing beads and bangles, long shirts and long skirts and in sandals and, of course, carrying anti-war signs. Everyone came dressed that way. Almost everyone. I came dressed as a soldier.

Everyone booed and I played along, of course. These were friends, after all. Nonetheless, I wondered afterwards why no one inquired about why I'd served, why I hadn't been a protester like them. Was I a draftee or volunteer? And, what was it that I did in Vietnam? (They hadn't known of my service before this party.) Was it lack of interest on their part? Or were some wounds best left untouched?

The thing is, I was, back then in the 1960s, just like them. I, too, opposed the war. But dissent and thinking for yourself don't always take you down the same path, so I opposed the war but still found myself in harm's way. Considering the options and expectations for someone like me, the latter needn't have happened. Educated, middle-class whites like me could and did avoid service in Vietnam back then by moving to Canada, for example, or arranging a family exemption, or getting a doctor to diagnose you as "gay," or contacting a congressman and letting him or her try to finesse an alternative assignment or deferment.

So why, after more than 40 years, do I revisit all that, let alone write a book? How many times can the same story be told? By way of an answer, I'll start with an e-mail I received out of the blue not long after that party. It was from a stranger in California who didn't know me; we'd never met. She was writing, she said, as a first generation Vietnamese American, to thank me for my military service. Her family, who had fled Vietnam after the fall of Saigon in 1975, had told her stories of the American effort to save their nation from

Communism. Recently, going over her elderly grandfather's papers, she'd come across my name. Seeing that I'd been one of those Americans, she'd felt moved to track me down and e-mail me just to say thank you.

From that prod, I couldn't help revisiting my Vietnam experience; which, in turn, prompted my wife to revisit her former prods that I tell my story. She had for years encouraged me to write my story, the whole story, not just the few articles I'd once sent to a magazine. And she knew my story well; she'd read most of my letters home, as most were addressed to her. (We were engaged at the time.) Your story is so different from the others, she'd insisted. Now, with seven grandchildren who'd otherwise never know what their Poppy saw and did in that war, I came around to her point of view. She was right. My story would be different.

But how different could it be from those standard Vietnam War narratives of books and movies, all those memoirs? These are the differences; I was a war-protester who did not burn his draft card or leave the country. When it was my turn to go, I went. I didn't grouse or agonize over it. And when I went over, I did my duty, which involved nothing brave or heroic; I was rarely in danger. There was nothing of high adventure, high jinx, or high drama. Any clashes I experienced that were memorable, and there were many, were variations of a culture clash, not an armed clash. When I was shaken up, and I often was, it was by culture shock, not combat stress.

Nor did I feel angry or bitter upon returning home. I brought home no nightmares or bad memories other than those of normal frustration and occasional embarrassment. I brought home neither scars nor disabilities nor memories of indulgence or excess. I brought home no remorse. What I did bring home were recollections of sometimes insights into other people and myself, systems of government, and familiar and unfamiliar customs; memories of difficult-to-justify dissatisfactions and hard-to-explain satisfactions; and memories of disconcerting attitudes and behaviors on my part. As a doctor I brought home memories of professional fulfillment that would never be repeated. I never stopped drawing on these or learning from them.

I used no street drugs over there and didn't use any back here, either. I just came home and picked up my civilian life where I'd left off, the same person, except, perhaps, wiser in some ways of the world, and about some of the agendas of people in the world, including my own. In all these ways my story would be different from the familiar Vietnam War story we've all become accustomed to.

There's more. I went over as a U.S. Army doctor — a healer, not a warrior — whose military mission it was, in uniform and in wartime, to take care of civilians. My military job, in other words, was civic-action related, not combat related, and it was for this reason that those occasional soldiers I did treat came to me for sickness, never war wounds, and, aside from rare exceptions were enemy soldiers, North Vietnamese and Vietcong (VC). How was this possible? It was possible because my medical chain of command, remarkably, terminated at the office of the South Vietnamese Ministry of Health, not somewhere in the U.S. Army Medical Corps. Mine was a State Department program, not a U.S. Army program. There had never been a program quite like this.

And this, too. Several years after my return to civilian life it became obvious that my program's mission, the MILPHAP counter-insurgency mission that, to this date, no one seems to have heard of, hadn't measured up to expectations, as if the South Vietnamese government's sending foreign troops into the lives of the people, into their faces, to fix problems they, the government, had identified, might not have been the optimal way to win back the people's flagging trust, affection, and loyalty. In the end, America gave up and pulled out and Saigon fell and the insurgents won and the Communists took over. But my contribution, what my team and I did — what all the MILPHAP teams had done serving that counter-insurgency mission — remained in my mind neither diminished nor invalidated. In any event, and at the very least, nobody died in Vietnam on my account or my team's account.

This book is directed to my grandchildren and their generation — actually anyone born after 1952, the last birth year of Americans subject to military draft. It is meant to ensure that there is a place on the shelf for this *other* kind of Vietnam War story, the story of something gained, not just lost, the story that what we mean by progress is never about preserving harmony; it's about destroying harmony and then restoring it. But, in real life, progress is sometimes less about the successful recovery of that lost harmony than about resilience in the face of its loss. Finally, this book is about the discovery that a humbling experience can, over time, actually enlighten and satisfy. I came to appreciate over time, to my surprise, relief, and chagrin, not that we're all human, but that, I'm only human. Maybe, as a nation, we've edged a bit closer to acceding that we're just "one among many."

I use the terms *culture shock* and *culture clash* to describe what appear to be ordinary human interactions because they best capture their impact on me and help give perspective to my unorthodox medical practice, even though not all were obviously related to cultural factors. I thought about them this way because that helped me absolve the other person of anything personal or malicious, an advantage when processing thorny ethical issues. And so I came to feel more chagrin and embarrassed than irked and angry, more inclined to examine and try to understand, than to become impatient and look to blame. It made it easier to seek ways to accept, even accommodate. And, while there may have been offense given and taken, there was never violence. I've not tried to connect the dots, however, from these examples of culture shock to those egregious forms of interpersonal interaction — again, among colleagues and allies — that, in contrast, did result in violence. Who has not heard of My Lai or "fragging," iconic of this latter phenomenon, now iconic of the Vietnam War (or of "insider attacks," theirs and ours, a later Afghanistan variant)? Who hasn't read about sexual abuse and the high suicide rate among returning war veterans? Could those be the same thing only of different intensity and with a tipping point where "shock" advances to "clash," a clash that occurs with one's own self as well as with one's mates? Or might those reflect a character flaw, possibly brain-injury driven, that predisposes an individual to violence or to intolerable vulnerability? In which case, are we talking about a soldier's low anger-threshold? Or low pain-threshold? Is the relevant impulse principally one of violence, towards hurting or controlling another, or towards relieving oneself of intolerable fear or pain or unbearable mental commotion?

Now, this caution. My account includes oversimplifications of some complicated political and historical events in addition to an inevitable author bias. About the former, I found that in writing this account, it was only by virtue of oversimplification that I was able to grasp and view the complex and nuanced historical narrative of Vietnam and the war. Oversimplifications, of course, always leave something out and mislead. But there are times when, like now, a story's merit in helping a reader get a handle on confusing material compensates for whatever is left out or off target. About author bias, I opt to leave my bias in place. Where I am able, I shall try to account for its being there in the first place. It seems too much the soul of this account to be unceremoniously erased away. Readers deserve to know *its* history, too.

The following were (and are) my biases. I have an abhorrence for coercion and injustice and betrayal of trust. Also, I don't like bullies, foreign or domestic. I believe American foreign policy should be transparently anchored in a national interest and believe, furthermore, that moral leadership is in our national interest. The litmus test for what is or is not in our national interest, for me, is whether or not, at our American "village" level — our "Joe Six-Pack" level — average Americans are able to connect the dots. I believe that we should help an ally in a quid pro quo arrangement to repel a foreign invader. I believe that we should *not* help that same ally repel internal dissidents.

Which brings us to the grey area of Vietnam in the 1960s. Here it appeared that one nation, North Vietnam, was exporting aggression and subversion — stirring up dissent — in a neighbor nation and ally of ours, South Vietnam. The North denied doing this or justified it. But, here's the thing. Was South Vietnam even a "nation" back then? Was it even empowered to enter into a treaty with us? Or with anyone? The Geneva Accords of 1954, which we insisted over and over be adhered to, say no. The Geneva Accords, according to some, say that South Vietnam was merely one-half of a country, arbitrarily and temporarily severed from its other half, making two regrouping "zones" (as some described them at the time), with the South administered by an appointed head, not an elected leader, of a caretaker government that was specifically enjoined from making an alliance with any nation, pending reunification. Then, again, America didn't sign those accords (even as it held North Vietnam accountable to them). Then, again, if South Vietnam really was a nation that raises the question of whether our military involvement was even legal under our Constitution. Congress never declared war.

Finally, and given these questions, here's one more question. Are my personal leanings or preferences in this matter even "biases"? Couldn't they be considered interpretations or opinions? Was it bias, for example, that many in America at that time called our post–1965 buildup of American combat forces on the ground, "McNamara's War," inasmuch as Secretary of Defense Robert McNamara was the principal policy-maker behind this not-officially-war war? Arguably, the term "McNamara's War" was as much an informed interpretation as a bias, no? (Then, again, back in 1952, didn't President Truman promote the American Legation in Saigon to embassy status, and didn't that mean South Vietnam *was* a sovereign country?)

You get the point. Let's just begin.

In the chapters to follow, the paragraphs in italics were taken directly from personal communications, mainly letters written home 1966–67. The voice in these letters is the voice of a young man, age 27 to 29.

1

Backgrounds: Theirs, Ours and Mine

A Summary History of the Vietnamese People and Attempts by Others to Control Them, 208 BCE–1950 CE

The Vietnamese people were originally the Yueh, named for their home of origin, an autonomous kingdom comprising the north of today's Vietnam and a southern portion of China (today's Kwang-tung Province). In 208 BCE it had already been, for several centuries, home to a flourishing Bronze Age culture. It was annexed by China in 111 CE and, for most of the next millennium until 939, was governed as a Chinese province. Then came the fall of the Chinese T'ang dynasty. In the unrest that followed, Chinese rule over this kingdom was overthrown. The influence of the Chinese culture on the Vietnamese people, apart from language, proved durable and permanent. Equally permanent was the resentment that Vietnamese people subsequently felt towards any foreign control.

Over the course of time the Vietnamese people's name and place-name, Yueh and Yueh-nan ("south of Yueh"), were transformed into Viet and Vietnam ("distant south"), as they expanded southward along the eastern rim of the Indochina peninsula, pushing from one small rice-bearing delta on into the next, expanding their wet-rice economy. The Vietnamese intermingled with, annexed, sometimes fought with and displaced into the highlands, or assimilated into their numbers, other peoples they encountered who had been there ahead of them. Because some invaders from the sea, like some of the peninsula's aboriginal inhabitants, likewise retreated or were pushed into the central highland plateau areas and mountains, that region eventually became home to a variety of peoples whose racial, religious, and linguistic roots can today be traced not only to India to the west and Tibet and Mongolia to the

7

north, but also to the Austro-Indonesia lands to the east and south. Vietnam today recognizes 54 distinct ethnic minorities.

For brief periods the Vietnamese were united as a people, but most of the time they were fighting one another. When French Roman Catholic missionaries appeared on the scene in the 17th century, which was a full century after European traders first appeared, the Vietnamese people, headquartered in Hue, had only recently taken serious command of the Mekong Delta from the Khmer (Cambodian) people living there. The subsequent trade with the French and evangelization by missionaries had a momentous impact on the life and culture of the Vietnamese people, especially in the southernmost part, such as the introduction of Western systems of government, education, and transportation along with a Latin-based script.

In the 19th century things changed. Like other European powers at that time, France, with its revolution and Napoleonic Wars behind it, began looking towards the Orient with expansionist intentions, not just trading interests. Paradoxically, this expansionist impulse corresponded to the opposite impulse for the Vietnamese emperors of that time, who were beginning to look inward. The latter's emerging isolationist spirit led, eventually, to a condemnation of the presence of foreign missionaries. (Christianity and Confucianism, one element of this tension, offer quite different visions of the individual's relationship to the state.) In 1858, following a particularly egregious period of persecution of Christian missionaries, the French military stepped in. There was resistance, but by 1884, not only the Vietnamese but all the peoples of Indochina were under French control. The Southeast Asian peninsula became "French" Indochina.

Vietnam, which composed the eastern part of French Indochina, was viewed as three distinct territories or "countries" of Vietnamese people. There was the southernmost part, Cochin China.[1] The inhabitants of this, the most recently settled and most underdeveloped in terms of traditional social structure and institutions, would become the most "French" of the three. The part farthest to the north, which abutted the Vietnamese people's home of origin in China, was called Tonkin. The middle section, including the imperial capital, Hue, was Annam (or An-nam). (Permitting Hue to keep its emperor enabled the French to facilitate these assignments.) The borders of Laos and Cambodia, along with Vietnam, were also delineated.

These three Vietnamese entities of Indochina were, by the end of the 19th century, under nearly total French control. Anti-colonial resistance to all this, of course, was present almost from the start. But as Bernard Fall observed, "50 years of French administration were about to begin, a short span in comparison to the 1,000 years of Chinese occupation that Viet-Nam had known earlier. But in terms of their impact upon Viet-Nam's future, those 50 years proved as fateful as the full 1,000."[2] For some, however, this meant progress and was welcomed. This was especially the case in Saigon, the capital of what would come to be known as the "mercantile" south.

Those indigenous people for whom the central mountains and highlands of Indochina were now home, people who bristled at any outsider efforts to take them over, continued to be left alone. Overall, the rice-planting lowland peoples on both sides of the Indochina peninsula, the Cambodian kings, for example, and the Vietnamese kings, preferred leaving these indigenous tribes in place as a buffer between them. The French, likewise, found this arrangement acceptable and continued it, and in exchange for keeping the lowlanders out the French were allowed a free hand in establishing for themselves plantations of coffee and rubber in the highlands. The Vietnamese accepted a symbolic tribute but otherwise left the tribes to themselves, a relationship that continued until 1954. These mountain tribes (known today as the Thuong ethnic minority) were introduced to the Western world by their French moniker, *Montagnard*, or "mountaineer." I will use the term *Montagnard* for consistency.

In 1940 the French Vichy government permitted Japanese troops to enter Vietnam. Starting in December 1941, Vietnam, now a puppet regime of Vichy Frenchmen, became a virtual colony of Japan. An independence movement, the Communist-led Vietnam Independence League ("Vietminh"), was organized to resist this. In early 1945 the Japanese granted Vietnam its independence, under Japanese "protection," of course. Its capital was Hanoi. (Cochin China was not included in this entity.)

The terms of the Japanese surrender to the Allies in 1945 obliged the Japanese to transfer the power they'd assumed in Vietnam over to the Vietminh, the best-armed, -led, and -organized of the several competing nationalist contenders. Provisional government status was given to this now "independent" Vietnam entity, headed by Ho Chi Minh. However, at war's end, to muddy the waters, the non–Communist Chinese Koumintang army of Chiang Kai-shek, America's wartime ally and the Vietnamese people's longtime neighbor and former ruler, moved south into Tonkin ostensibly to disarm the Japanese 21st Division. This meant that Ho had to deal with the Chinese first. (Looting seemed foremost on the Chinese agenda.) The good news for Ho was that the freedom of movement of the French would now be limited to the south. So Ho Chi Minh signed off on a *modus vivendi* with France that mollified France because it provided little independence in the south but, more important, effected the Chinese departure and bought time for Ho to consolidate his position in the north.

Many expected that America would support this new reality, this provisional Vietnamese government in the north headed by Ho. After all, during

World War II President Roosevelt repeatedly advocated postwar independence for colonial peoples. But President Truman had another concern, containing Russia with NATO, and this meant a strong France.

French admiral Georges D'Argenlieu, copying the Vietminh strategy in the north, sponsored the creation of the Provisional Government of Cochin China with former Emperor Bao Dai at its head, but the Hanoi-based "independent" Vietnam already in place (the Democratic Republic of Vietnam) promptly declared Cochin China as under *its* jurisdiction. Ho knew that three-fifths of French holdings in Indochina were concentrated in rice-rich Cochin China, that the French owned two-thirds of the rice plus all the mines, all the shipping, and virtually all the industry and nearly all the banks, and that the rubber plantations, despite the war, had never had to stop operations. He knew, too, that, behind their ostensible crusade to stop Communism, the French really envisioned Cochin China as a sort of future permanent French puppet state. However, before politicians could address this conundrum, violence erupted.

What followed was the French Indochina War. More than a few of the parties involved had difficulty determining who, exactly, their primary enemy was. For the Vietnamese, was it still the French seeking to reestablish their colony? Or was it the Communist-dominated Vietminh? Or the Communist Chinese army of Mao Zedong across the border? (Chiang Kai-shek and his Nationalist Army had, by now, withdrawn from Tonkin and, by 1949, been forced off mainland China and onto the island of Formosa.) More than a few would change sides in this conflict.

From Financial Assistance to the French to Advisors to Vietnamese on Reform: American Involvement, 1950–1963

By 1950, Russia had exploded its first atomic bomb, China had become Communist, and Communist North Korea had invaded South Korea. America, in response to the latter, sent a military mission with advisors to help the French who were insisting (disingenuously, according to many) that the French interest had now shifted from recovering their colonial property to a "crusade against Communism." That year the U.S. Military Assistance Advisory Group (MAAG), consisting of 35 men, arrived in Vietnam to train French troops receiving U.S. weapons in how to use them.

By 1953, America was subsidizing nearly 80 percent of the French costs of their Indochina War. (By 1954 the cost topped $2 billion.) It was as if America's determination that France be a reliable part of the evolving pre-

NATO European Defense Community fully trumped any interest the U.S. had in supporting nationalistic aspirations of the Vietnamese. The confident French did most of the fighting against the Communist Vietminh, whose strength primarily was in the north. "The Vietnamese Army," Phan Quang Dan, advisor to Bao Dai, lamented, "is without responsible Vietnamese leaders, without ideology, without objective, without enthusiasm, without fighting spirit, and without popular backing."[3] Bao Dai would soon begin spending more and more time away from his office and at one of his favorite retreats, his hunting lodge in Ban Me Thuot in the central highlands, where he was popular with the people and enjoyed elephant race spectacles.

President Harry Truman's policy of military containment of Communism, his Truman Doctrine, which had been articulated in 1947, had committed the United States, it seemed, to a course that now joined us to two unreconcilable allies, the indispensable but colonialist-tainted French and a weak and divided Vietnamese people. An uncomplicated sound-bite to this unfolding Indochina foreign policy, coined by President Eisenhower, became popular at the time. It was the "falling domino theory." If one Southeast Asian country fell to Communism, the theory warned, all the others, Cambodia, Thailand, Burma, Malaysia, India, Indonesia, and the Philippines, would topple as well, like a row of dominoes. And then came the total French defeat at their self-proclaimed impregnable stronghold at Dien Bien Phu in Tonkin near the Chinese border in 1954, a debacle that took everyone by surprise. (A desperate Arthur Radford, chairman of the Joint Chiefs of Staff, when defeat appeared inevitable, actually proposed that America make nuclear strikes against the Vietminh.) I was in high school at the time.

Thus it was that, in the spring of 1954 in Geneva, Switzerland, the international committee sitting to negotiate an armistice between North and South Korea bumped to the top of their agenda a ceasefire in Indochina. There was urgency. (There were three separate ceasefire accords; the other two covered Cambodia and Laos.) A key breakthrough was all parties agreeing to a temporary two-year partition of the country into a north and a south. The two parts would be separated at the 17th Parallel by a demilitarized zone (DMZ). There would be a 300-day window for the regrouping of forces and also for the movement of civilian populations to the zone of their choice. There would be a two-year pause before consultations between the two zones would begin, and that would lead to free general elections that would determine the preferred form of government of the reunified country. There would be a ban on the introduction of any "fresh troops, military personnel, arms, and munitions, or military bases" pending the outcome of those elections.

Bao Dai's government in the south now included his hand-picked selection for prime minister, Ngo Dinh Diem (phonetically, "Ziem"), an anti-

Communist with unique scholar-official credentials (i.e., a mandarin), who came on board a month after the Geneva meetings were underway and made a point of refusing to sign the accords.[4] Below the surface, simmering were the many other agendas. It was no surprise that the framers of the accord felt obliged, simply to move forward, to leave some details vague. One detail, however, was not vague. It was the proviso that ensured that the International Commission of Supervision and Control of Vietnam (ICC), consisting of Indian, Canadian, and Polish representatives, would have no police powers, and no power whatsoever to enforce any of the accord's provisions. (The subsequent unravelling of the Geneva Accords thus came as a surprise to no one.)

Elections were never held. As early as 1955 it became evident to Bao Dai, principally by virtue of Diem's egregious police methods and his unabashedly dictatorial inclinations, that he'd appointed the wrong man premier. Bao Dai annulled Diem's powers and dismissed him. In response, Diem, quickly calling for a referendum, not only replaced Bao Dai but also proclaimed himself South Vietnam's first president, prime minister, defense minister, and supreme commander of the armed forces, which meant that Diem now had more powers to control the country (South Vietnam) administratively and politically than had been held by the French governors general in years past. Further, "despite the fact that the earlier Vietnamese Emperors ruled by divine right, the Presidential powers as prescribed in the Constitution of the Republic of Vietnam, which was promulgated in October 1956, were broader and more all-encompassing than those the Emperors wielded in practice."[5]

Still, the United States sent aid to the Diem government, holding out hope that, as repeatedly requested, Diem would actually institute the increasingly critical social and economic reforms necessary to bring people into his camp. Eqbal Ahmad, professor at the School of Labor and Industrial Relations at Cornell, a Pakistani citizen and anti-war activist, set it out plainly. It was "morbid optimism," he wrote, "to expect an absentee aristocrat [Diem] to supplant a leader [Ho] who had devoted a lifetime to the liberation of his country, and to defeat a leadership and cadres whose organic ties with the peasants were cemented by the bitter struggle for independence."[6]

Unfortunately, Diem's focus was never on the reforms his American advisors were urging but rather on consolidating his own power which, in a weird way, was in line with the American tendency to view Communism, as war historian Marvin Gettleman, put it, "as an evil so monstrous that *any measures taken to suppress it are justified*" (italics mine).[7] The result: people in the villages not only fell silent, they began lending their assistance to the Communist insurgents, even taking up arms at their side. The government we were supporting was, as we stood by, becoming progressively more detested and discredited. Those long-overdue reforms were now imperative. It was in this context, in 1960, the year of a failed coup against Diem, that the Communists in South Vietnam formed a National Liberation Front to include non–Communists in their insurgency. They called themselves "Vietcong."

In 1962, a Military Assistance Command, Vietnam (MACV), was created to augment the MAAG advisory group, which had, by then, significantly expanded in reaction to the expanding presence of Vietminh, and, more recently, Vietcong, in South Vietnam. MACV quickly become MAAG's supervisor. The MAAG U.S. military forces now numbered 3,200. MACV headquarters was installed in Saigon. (Three years later I would be called up to join that MACV group.) In late 1963, the Hanoi leadership began to formally commit units of the North Vietnamese Army (NVA) to assist the fighting in the South. The time of advisors was passing. The time for direct American involvement was at hand. The finger-pointing was ratcheting up. Accusations mounted over which side was bringing in the most troops.

In 1963, the command of the Special Forces, the Green Berets, passed from the U.S. Embassy, where it had begun, to MACV. These were the paramilitary forces initially sponsored by the U.S. Mission (Embassy) that recruited from Montagnard tribes in the Central Highlands. Because Montagnards were obvious targets for Communist propaganda — their dissatisfaction with the Vietnamese government over its disrespectful, exploitative, and abusive treatment was no secret — here, as part of a Civilian Irregular Defense Group (CIDG) they could serve as a counterbalance to Vietcong infiltration into the porous central highlands. These soldiers were called "strikers" by the 12-man American teams that led them.[8]

The Tipping Point: From Advisors to Boots on the Ground, 1963–1965

The American secretary of state, Dean Rusk, now understood that it was not only necessary to get these reforms going, it was absolutely critical. It no longer appeared possible to oppose the Vietminh — now Vietcong — purely by military means, so the people's allegiance and contribution was a priority. But the people of South Vietnam were still caught between Communism, on the one hand, and something they couldn't accept, on the other. Before it was the French colonial regime. Now it was a type of dictatorship that was, in the words of Devillers, "at one and the same time fascist and medieval."[9]

The final straw was about a flag, a Buddhist flag, and the Buddha's birthday. In May 1963, according to David Halberstam's Pulitzer Prize–winning report, "It started with the Buddhists' wish to fly their flag in Hue on the

Buddha's birthday. The Government, citing an old regulation, replied that only Government flags were permitted in public. Thousands of Buddhists demonstrated and the Government broke up the demonstration by firing into the crowd killing nine."[10] The government subsequently refused to apologize or even acknowledge the facts, let alone offer reparations, and insisted, instead, that the nine fatalities died at the hands of the Vietcong. Diem's response to the delegations and protests of his countrymen was, according to witnesses, to treat them as nothing more than unpleasant affronts to his family. Protests spread.

The escalating war was now costing the United States $1.5 million a day. The U.S. Embassy leaned on Diem to settle the issue quickly. Dissent in the U.S. Senate was blunt. "I would have the United States get out of South Vietnam and save the American people the hundreds upon hundreds of millions of dollars that our Government is pouring down that rat hole," declared a disgusted Wayne Morse (D., Oregon).[11] The waves of protest in the United States were unparalleled in recent American history. When Mrs. Ngo Dinh Nhu dismissed the protests as merely evidence that the Buddhists had obviously been infiltrated by Communists, it wasn't just the embassy that was aghast. President Kennedy tactfully let it be known that, in his view, the Vietnamese people wouldn't be upset to see Diem go. On November 2 of that year, 1963, generals of South Vietnamese Army conducted a military coup d'état, which was followed by Diem's assassination. When, weeks later, President Kennedy was assassinated in Dallas, Texas (November 22, 1963), curiously absent from the list of suspected conspirators in his assassination was anyone remotely associated with the Diem family or even Southeast Asia.

Before the first year of President Johnson's administration was completed, frustrated as he must have been with the resistance our Vietnamese allies were putting forth to reforms, he got Congress to pass a resolution authorizing him to wage all-out war against North Vietnam without a formal declaration of war. This was the Tonkin Gulf Resolution, which followed an August 1964 Gulf of Tonkin "incident." Bombing of the north began later that year. In March the Marines landed and a sustained American bombing campaign of North Vietnam, Operation Rolling Thunder, was initiated.

During that first year of Johnson's presidency, Montagnards of the Central Highlands had reached a tipping point of their own. They took up arms against the ethnic Vietnamese, whom they saw now as their invaders, their occupiers. (Recalling that the resettlement of nearly a million civilian and ethnic Vietnamese refugees from the North into the South, after the partition following the 1954 Geneva Accords, was accomplished partly by relocating refugees in tribal lands. Subsequent forced relocation of rebellious peasants from the coastal plains into the highlands further aggravated that problem.)

Until early 1965, the war had been considered in Washington to be a civil war. A survey conducted the year before had shown that one-quarter of Americans didn't know there was any fighting going on in Vietnam at all, even though there were 23,000 American military personnel there. The fiction was that Americans were there but weren't fighting. They were, in large part, "advisors." In February 1965 (the month I received my notice from my local Draft Board to have an Armed Forces physical examination) a State Department publication, "Aggression from the North: The Record of North Vietnam's Campaign to Conquer South Vietnam," the so-called White Paper, was issued to make the case that the war was, and had been all along, the North's attempts to conquer the South. (It failed to make that case.)

President Johnson, it seemed, was running out of patience. He was desperate to force the North to the negotiating table. His offer of negotiations without preconditions appeared to reflect such a desperation. And yet, his one precondition, that he not negotiate with the Vietcong, suggested the opposite and proved to be the deal-breaker. Around this time Senator Barry Goldwater, regarded by some as a contender for the Republican nomination for the presidency, made the proposal that we start using low-yield atomic bombs.[12]

By that spring, 1965 (by which time I had passed my physical and had been offered a commission as lieutenant in the Army Reserves), the American anti-war movement was nationwide and gathering steam alongside the growing nationwide confusion about America's role in South Vietnam. There were marches and demonstrations in Washington, D.C., and a new form of protest, "teach-ins," at universities.

Frank Church (D., Idaho) summarized the predicament we'd created for ourselves succinctly: "We have come to treat 'Communism,' regardless of what form it may take in any given country, as the enemy. We fancy ourselves as guardian of the 'free' world, though most of it is not free and never has been. We seek to immunize this world against further Communist infection through massive injections of American aid, and, wherever necessary, through direct American intervention." Then, he pointed out obstacles to such action: "First, it exceeds our national capability; second, among the newly-emerging nations, where the specter of Western imperialism is dreaded more than Communism, such a policy can be self-defeating." He added, "For most Africans and Asians, our concept of self-government and individual freedom is totally unreal, having never been experienced. In many, if not most, of these emergent lands, it is Capitalism, not Communism, which is the ugly word."[13]

That June, my rank was advanced to captain and I was ordered to active duty. By the time I reported for duty that August our massive troop buildup had begun. I was assigned to MACV Headquarters, Saigon.

America of the 1950s

Throughout the 1950s the "domino" or "falling domino" theory held sway, firmly joined to our American self-image, which was, in my view, not only seductive and addicting but blinding as well. We felt, in essence, that we could possess everything we touched and fix anything we broke. We were number one and the people of the world loved and admired us for this, even though this made it clear to them that, in our eyes, they could never amount to more than second best. Having never lost a war, we seemed destined to prevail in any contest.

So profound and malignant was this self-image and its accompanying self-deception that it couldn't help but color our foreign policy. With the image of Communism as not just the enemy but evil, there came the obligation to fight it, not just as a quest to keep the world free, but as a moral imperative. These ideas were joined to the certainty that America would prevail. As a result, the facts took a hit. The media often saw this disconnect and suspected our government was lying with its upbeat pronouncements and predictions. But, looking back, it seemed that the government leaders and spokespersons weren't lying. They believed what they were saying because they simply believed what *they* were being told, and it was not uncommon for them to be told what it was believed they wanted to hear. So we believed, too. Most of us. This business had to be done for the good of the world and we had to do it. Why? Because we could.

Meanwhile, our own domestic "liberation" movements, such as nuclear disarmament, women's liberation, the sexual revolution, and the civil rights movement — all of these wake-up calls — always seemed, in the 1950s, anyway, to include a snooze-alarm option. By pushing that snooze-alarm button we were able to return to our preferred reality, what one could call our dream-world. How else are we to understand why, given the Vietnamese imperative to rid themselves of colonizers and occupiers and everything in between, we nonetheless kept edging farther and farther out along that slippery slope? It was as if that Vietnamese imperative provided them with grease as well as grit.

During those years, the 1950s, I went from a pre-adolescent to a college graduate. My memories of that time include the appearance of the polio vaccine. It came out too late for me to enjoy seeing movie matinees with their cliff-hanger movie serials. Crowds were a great risk factor for this contagious disease, exposure to which put you at risk for a life in an iron lung. My parents had both been youngsters during the influenza pandemic of years before and were resolved to take no chances with their children. So, I never saw those cliff-hanger movie serials. The polio vaccine made movie theaters safe; that's what it meant to me. And I remember reading about Rosa Parks refusing to give up her seat on a bus in Montgomery, Alabama, because she was the sort of underdog I admired. In her own way and on her own terms she "stood up" to her enemies. Of course I understood that I looked like her enemies, but that wasn't the point. From that moment on whenever I thought of Rosa Parks I was black like her.

A Rocky Start to the Sixties

At the start of the 1960s our sense of the world and our place in it was still dominated by the urgency to contain the spread of Communism. I was a medical student at the Albert Einstein College of Medicine in Bronx, New York, and remember the showdown between President Kennedy and the Soviets over their placing missiles in Cuba that were aimed at us. I refused to believe that that would lead to war; that's how strong my denial was, how scary it was. I couldn't even let myself process that possibility, that reality. I kept telling myself, it's like a competition; our missiles in Turkey are aimed at them. Now they've caught up and have some in our neighborhood aimed at us. Tit for tat. Just like a game.

I remember exactly where I was and what I was doing when I learned that Kennedy had been shot in Dallas, Texas. I was visiting my parents in New Haven, Connecticut. At the moment the news broke I was driving to pick up my mother from an appointment. Again, I couldn't believe what I was hearing. I was sure the reports were mistaken, that he was just fine. That's how unnerving it was, those unreal moments of suspense, waiting for news from Dallas over the radio.

My Objections to an American War

If I was apolitical, why was I anti-war? I had three reasons. The first had to do with fear and distrust. I distrusted the military. Maybe it was something President Eisenhower had said about the military and that my father repeated. In any event, since my early teens when I'd first heard their pitch about hating and fearing Communism, deep down I wouldn't let it compute. I knew that if America used a nuclear weapon Russia would retaliate. And, if they knew we knew this, why wouldn't they strike preemptively? So, I never let myself connect Communism to my world, to me. My teachers made it easy. In lessons about Communism in high school, the propagandistic tone of the articles presented to us as academic material was insulting — as if my classmates and I couldn't handle the facts and be trusted with the truth. That made it easy to dismiss the messengers. My take away-lesson was always less about the image of Communism that was being pitched at me than it was about the image of myself that was reflected back at me as the catcher of that stuff. I looked stupid. I looked untrustworthy and easily manipulated. In later conversations, explanations of why America was supporting the Vietnamese cause it always came out sounding more like reasons the *Vietnamese* were supporting *our* cause. In any event, there were just not enough dots for me to be able, let alone willing, to take what was happening somewhere in Southeast Asia and connect it to me. My fear-plate was already full to overflowing with the dread of Russia dropping an A-bomb on us.

Perhaps, as an American and aware of our national narrative of expelling our colonizer, Great Britain, and subsequent sympathy for all underdogs, I deliberately turned a blind eye to the likelihood that South Vietnam, population 14.5 million, after winning its independence from France after 90 years as a colony, would allow itself to become a puppet of Russia and international Communism. But even if I wasn't in denial and allowed myself to imagine Vietnam and all Southeast Asia becoming a puppet of Soviet imperialism, I still couldn't see how that would compel Russia to attack America with an A-bomb.

My second reason was emotional. It had to do with my aversion to apocalyptic, grandiose pronouncements of any kind — in this example, Free World versus Evil. I knew American history. I knew about the role of internal repression, rapacity, and racism, not only on the part of individuals and groups but also of national policy, and of external subversion of other nations' governments — brutal and murderous — in the pursuit of our nation's narrative. I became especially turned off by the unabashed use of the word, *crusade* in pronouncements relating to Communism. I may not have known my world politics but I knew my world history. If the Crusades of history taught us anything, it was that the collateral damage that accompanies such a "holy" enterprise brings shame to would-be crusaders that is everlasting.

My third reason was practical. There were simply too many Asian Communists over there in Asia for us Americans to handle, let alone beat into submission, let alone convert to our form of government. The numbers, alone, ruled out any chance of my supporting an American war there. What would we do, occupy China?

Caught in the Draft

In April 1965, when I received my draft notice, I was a doctor, 27 years old, unmarried, and finishing my medical internship at the Long Island College Hospital in Brooklyn, New York. I'd been preparing to begin my specialty training in psychiatry at Yale in New Haven, Connecticut, that summer. Of course I knew there was trouble in Vietnam, a country somewhere in Asia. At that time I was apolitical. Also, anti-war.

Having an aversion to things military (an issue of trust, not pacifism), I had, in my attempt to defer being drafted until I'd completed my specialty training, applied to the only uniformed service that wasn't military, the Public Health Service (PHS). I'd applied to their Berry Plan in my final year of medical school, late for such an application. Why late? Because I didn't want to think about it. Because of this delay, by the time the letter arrived inviting me to come to Washington, D.C., for an interview, I'd already graduated medical school in Bronx, New York, and had moved on to start my internship in Brooklyn, never notifying the PHS of my change of address. When I finally remembered and called to check the status of my application, they told me they'd already sent out the invitation and, not hearing from me, assumed I'd lost interest and moved on. I was available to the draft.

The letter came in February 1965, from Selective Service Local Board No. 9 in New Haven, Connecticut, directing me to have an Armed Forces physical examination prior to my being allocated to the army, navy, or air force. I passed that exam and that April was offered a commission as first lieutenant in the army reserves. If I declined this offer (an offer others declined to accept and later regretted) I would have been promptly re-drafted as an enlisted man. So I became a first lieutenant. In July I was notified that my rank had been advanced to captain and I was ordered to active duty. My assignment was to Headquarters, U.S. Military Assistance Command, Vietnam (MACV). I was to depart for Vietnam November 4.

My reaction was a sick, sinking sensation because I'd seen this coming, followed by embarrassment. Why embarrassment? Because I should have been able to defer the draft if not outright avoid it. Being caught like this, my mind, signified I'd messed up, and I had, by applying late to the Berry Plan. I hadn't been paying attention. But then came relief. Why relief? Because after so many stressful years on the treadmill of uninterrupted medical studies and training, pushing myself, I needed a break and, deep down, recognized that this might turn out to be just that break.

I did not tell anyone about these considerations, emotions, and that screw-up. My family and friends, rallying to give me support, had enough to handle with their own emotions. They wanted to help, of course. They all wanted to show me how to get this order rescinded. How could I tell them I needed the break? Let alone that it was my fault and open up *that* can of worms? So I listened to their advisories and strategies and commiseration and kept my counsel, which wasn't difficult because I was that kind of person. I was private and never much into sharing deepest feelings, those I was aware of, anyway. Keeping my counsel had a long history, too, if a sometimes flawed track record. I'd been that way since childhood. How ironic, I remember thinking to myself, that I should be taking my break and reaching for sanctuary in a war zone and on the other side of the world. (And how sad, too, looking back now, that being called upon to serve one's country should be counted, even for a brief moment, as a blot on one's record, a failure or fault of some kind.)

Who Was I, Anyway?

I was born in New Haven, Connecticut, in 1938 to a middle-class, white, Jewish family; mother a teacher, father a physician. I was a second son and middle child. At the time of my draft notice I'd never been west of Ohio. I'd studied but never learned to speak a foreign language. I'd worked summers and vacations since I was 14 (and six feet tall) as a mail sorter at the post office, a hospital orderly, a camp counsellor for emotionally disturbed children. I'd worked on a road gang laying sewer pipe and as a deck hand on clam boats and a harbor dredge. I'd played sports with boys in the neighborhood but I wasn't good; I was usually picked toward the middle. I liked basketball but couldn't jump so I shot baskets alone or with my brother or played pick-up games in our driveway. I played no organized sport until college when I rowed on the crew, but that was only by default. Crew was the only college sport where having no prior experience was preferred; no bad habits to unlearn, the coach told me.

The noteworthy features of my childhood and adolescence, for the purpose of this account, were my habits of working hard that got me into and through college and medical school, and the habit of being trusting and well behaved. I was probably what would be called an over-achiever. I was dutiful and obedient and I strove as I did because that was what was expected of me. I pushed myself to get ahead because that was what I was supposed to do. To fail and fall behind, when I was very young and my father away in the war, was linked in my mind and gut to an irrational fear of being left behind and abandoned. I might point out that, like the parents of others of my generation, my parents had endured the Great Depression and made sacrifices, both then and in wartime. My father, at age 37 and a doctor and no longer subject to the draft, enlisted and served two years aboard a navy attack transport that brought troops to beachheads for amphibious landings and then treated the wounded afterwards. At war's end, he lived away from home some additional years to train in a specialty he'd practiced on-the-fly aboard ship, reconstructive surgery. All told, my dad was mostly absent from my life while I was from five to eleven years old.

Back then, when parents spoke, we children listened. Some might point out that ours was the generation that lived in the shadow of nuclear war, meaning that it was a time of denial and sustained, albeit contained, existential anxiety. We grew up in the shadow of annihilation. I was a quiet child, slow to anger, easy to like. I wasn't tough or daring. When our generation was dubbed the "silent" generation I neither saw nor took offense. Rocking the boat or pushing the envelope that was the status quo, inasmuch as it would have entailed rocking my parents boat and pushing *their* envelope, would have seemed to me the ultimate in selfish ingratitude, the ultimate of disrespect to the War Generation. They'd sacrificed, starved and bled for those "boats" and "envelopes." Thus, when my turn came to be "me," to "do my own thing" (expressions that were not even in our lexicon back then), I intuitively understood that it would have to be much later and somewhere else. It wouldn't be in their faces.

So how did we boys manifest and deal with our emotional "baggage" (another term not yet in our lexicon)? We managed by denying we carried emotional baggage, or that we carried emotions at all. We played it "cool." We were "cool," or tried to be, and we practiced this by denial and by redirecting all the potentially risky passions. I still recall the movies of the 1940s and 50s with their set-pieces in which a grown man, prodded to say "I love you," would squirm and stammer. How else does one explain how we managed to avoid noticing, on my college campus, anyway, that there were refugees from an anti–Communist revolution in Hungary? How else did we manage not to pay attention to those former ROK (Republic of Korea) officers who came to study after the Korean War Armistice just two years earlier? I might have asked them, What happened? What did you do? How and why did you come here? But my pals and I preferred channelling our nervous tensions, hormonal energies, and other passions to football games and dating. Here, at least, battles were all play anyway, and outcomes could mean everything or nothing depending on your attitude. And we were "cool."

There was, of course, a down side to being "cool." Being cool took effort. That meant seeing certain things while managing, at the same time, not to notice or think about them. Our black swimmers didn't accompany teammates for swim meets in the Deep South. Colleges there wouldn't allow them in the pool, and Yale conceded. There were no campus protests. (Our biggest street protest in New Haven was over an ice-cream truck.) I'd been admitted to Yale under a quota, a limit for Jews. I felt lucky. Shouldn't I have felt indignant? But by graduation in 1959, a blitz was coming, and we should have seen it coming, and I'm not referring to mini-skirts, Hare Krishna, or LSD, which we took in stride. We — middle class whites as a class — weren't paying attention.

As I said, President Johnson had, several months earlier — this was March 1965 — initiated a bombing campaign of North Vietnam. The anti-war movement, of which I was a non-activist member, took exception and, later that year, a crowd of 45,000 would march in Washington in protest. Before I even reported for duty at Fort Sam Houston, San Antonio, Texas, that August, Congress had given its approval for troops on the ground in Vietnam, the Marines had landed, and a major call-up was underway. To complicate the picture on the ground in South Vietnam, there had recently begun, that second kind of insurgency wherein the Montagnards of the central highlands, many of whom had fought with the French at Dien Bien Phu, rose up. In September 1964 there was violence. I repeat all this because it was all unforeseen while, ironically, predictable in hindsight; and the eruption resonated eerily with one of our own. That summer of 1965 the Watts section of Los Angeles, a black minority community, erupted in riots and violence. (That's the blitz I was referring to earlier.)

Now comes the biggest irony. I had failed an examination during my internship and would have to make it up. (I did.) But why did I fail that exam? It was for lack of study. I simply wasn't interested enough to keep pushing myself at studies anymore. I was beat and had other interests. Truth be told, my interest in medicine was, and always had been, tempered by a more powerful interest in people, especially people like me, fictitious or real, who were ordinary and quiet but, when called upon, dared and explored and fought the dragon and had adventures. My choice of reading was, as long as I can remember, guided by this draw. It was true in college where I chose as my major Culture and Human Behavior, and it was true throughout medical school, where I always found a patient's story more compelling than his or her particular vital signs or lab results. On entering into internship, the mystery and details of how someone got to where he or she was continued to have the same value for me as the mystery and details of their illness. I had been following my bliss, in Joseph Campbell's terms, and it had caused me to stumble on my journey into a medical practice. But that stumble turned into a leap forward. That's the irony.

I'll explain. I'd known for years, and for many reasons, and on multiple levels, that this passion of mine would eventually lead me from general medicine into psychiatry. That academic failure I'd just mentioned hadn't been my first. (My left brain in those years, with its demand for logical precision and scientific rigor, had long and painfully and unsuccessfully struggled for dominance over my right brain's persistent non-rational sensibilities. I remember friends from medical school who I'd encountered years later telling me they remembered me as "the one who never smiled.") So it looked as if, for now, having been drafted, that specialty was on hold. But it only appeared to be on hold, because I was about to take an intercultural field trip. My final military destination was not going to be MACV Headquarters in Saigon but rather somewhere the central highlands, where I would be providing medical care to, among others, that same tribe that staged the Montagnard insurrection, the Rhade (E'De), along with their recent neighbors, those North Vietnamese refugees who'd been resettled in their front yard during the population transfers following the Geneva Accords of 1954.

But that was yet to come. For now, my destination was Headquarters, U.S. Military Assistance Command, Vietnam (MACV).

2

Citizen-Soldiering

The Big Buildup

As officer recruits we experienced perks and comfort and were made to feel important. The troop buildup was underway. In September 1965, the number of U.S. military in Vietnam reached 125,000. By December it would climb to 180,000, and General Westmorland would ask for another 250,000 over the coming year. When I completed my basic training in October of 1965, the monthly draft quota had gone up from 17,000 in August to 27,400 in September. That October it reached 36,000 and McNamara was predicting that the number of U.S. killed-in-action would be 1,000 a month. This buildup had its counterpart in the buildup we felt in our own importance, capacities, and expectations as doctor-officers. Just months out of internships, here we were taking crash courses in administering anesthesia and listening to lectures on brain surgery and abdominal surgery, identifying and distinguishing parasite eggs under a microscope, learning where to shoot in an ambush, and how to cope with casualties of biological, chemical, and nuclear warfare. Discreetly pernicious was the perception that we'd be filling in where there was an unfortunate lack of caregivers. We'd be Americans coming to the rescue. The reality, however, was that we were innocents expected to finesse a stacked deck.

Red Flags, Ours and a Timely Rank-Reversal

A dark side to both types of buildup, of troops and our self-importance, related to the effect military culture had on some of us and, conversely, the effect our civilian habits had on them. There was one occasion when a timely rank-reversal saved everyone's bacon.

In the first example a group of doctor-captains, out on bivouac one night, assaulted one of their own in their tent. True, the victim doctor-captain, the operational "company commander" in this exercise owing to prior ROTC experience, was obnoxious and provocative. But to require, in the morning, a medical evacuation by chopper to the hospital with broken ribs! How can such a thing be possible at the hands of educated men, professional men, licensed healers? Was it related to the abrupt transition from the responsible independence of civilian life to the culture of dependency, obedience, and control of a military culture with unexpected resonance with childhood memories of pretending and playtime? Was there a regressive pull towards an earlier, more immature developmental state vis-à-vis a "playmate's" infuriating behavior? But what about the self-correcting influence of reality-testing? We weren't children anymore. Had that been muted by the shift into this military culture? I think so.

I was remembering observing similar behavior among the teaching staff. We saw a film titled *1943* as an introduction to the concept of "civic action." The scenes showed black African people rounded up like cattle and pushed and shoved by white police. (It was about plague in Africa.) It showed DDT hoses unceremoniously pushed down blouses and pointed up dresses to spray this insecticide. The movie closed with this arresting comment by the narrator: "Sometimes the people don't seem to appreciate the wonderful good we're doing for them." Later, I raised my hand to point out the obvious disconnect, caregiving with disrespect. The colonel presenting this introduction to civic action erupted. "You tell them what's good for them!" he shouted in response. "And if they don't like it you arrest them and lock them up if you have to!" Everyone assumed he was joking and laughed. I was looking directly at him and he at me. He wasn't joking; he was out of control. When I pointed out that that behavior we'd just witnessed on film didn't seem likely to encourage acceptance of civic action he immediately rejoined, "The hell with civic action!" (My journal notes say only that he carried on in that vein a while before calming down. It was like a tantrum, a regressive moment.)

In the second example of civilian habits impacting on military ways, I was reprimanded by the colonel at Fort Bliss, where I'd been temporarily assigned dispensary duty while my team was being gathered. I'd struck a private soldier several times. Why? He'd come to sick call and appeared to be having a bout of what looked like uncontrollable hysterical "seizures." Nothing seemed to work, and I didn't want to knock him out with an injection of medication. So I did what I knew would work from my civilian training, even though it was not officially sanctioned in the military. I slapped him several times and the "seizures" stopped. I explained this to the colonel as a emergency medical intervention. (He accepted it.) Perhaps a better example is my listening to troopers' complaints without comment until they began to cry. It's what I learned in civilian training. There was, I remember, the trooper with a headache who appeared at sick call three days running. I told him his problem wasn't his headache. If he came in again he should be prepared to talk about what that might be. He did, and he did. He broke down. He was a country boy who broke horses for a living. He'd been isolated by fellow troopers. It seemed his lack of education and lack of resources for the cruel finesse of big city relationships made him an easy target. I made an appointment for him at Mental Health but he came back before it materialized. He'd taken an overdose of fiorinal, about 60 mg barbiturate-equivalent. He wanted out. His instinct said to escape, and he did what he could to effect that. He was subsequently separated from the service, diagnosis schizoid personality. He didn't have a schizoid personality disorder. He was a scared, overwhelmed, and depressed kid. (There'd be other occasions I'd question military psychiatric practice.)

Here's the example of rank-reversal. It was early 1966, and thousands of recruits were arriving each week. Some 250,000 American military men would be in or en route to South Vietnam by the coming spring. The base's dispensary space and doctor time was maxed out, and I was working 12-hour days. Influenza and strep throat were close to epidemic. Then a trooper died of spinal meningitis. Immediately, that soldier's barracks was put on quarantine status. Spinal meningitis strikes quickly, develops quickly, and spreads quickly. Our now augmented medical staff was on high alert. Stiff neck with forearm rash, unmistakable signs, meant evacuation to Beaumont Hospital and immediate medical attention. If caught in time it was treatable.

I was directed to make twice daily inspections at that deceased trooper's barracks. The lieutenant in command of the quarantined barracks had his troopers line up at attention by their bunks, two rows of 60 guys in undershorts and T-shirts. My first barracks inspection here turned out to be an embarrassing experience for me. I fully expected I'd take charge and conduct my kind of examination, but the lieutenant had his own plan, which he'd failed to mention to me. After I was introduced, I said to the lines of troopers, "At ease." No one moved. All remained stiffly at attention. I repeated, this time with more authority to my voice, "At ease!" Nothing. There I was, nonplussed and uncertain what to do next because I didn't understand what was happening. I couldn't get beyond the question of how to assess the presence of neck stiffness in 120 soldiers standing stiffly at attention. "This way, doctor," the lieutenant said quietly.

I followed him down the 1st row of soldiers, more concerned with appearances, with acting like I knew what I was doing and knew what was happening, than when and how I'd get to actually talk to these soldiers and properly examine them. But that changed dramatically when the first trooper I approached thrust out his arms at me, palms up — startling me, actually — followed by a head swivel in a tight circle. I got it! Flexible neck, no rash! *That* was the drill for this inspection! It was essentially a time-management exercise for optimal gain for the most people in the shortest time. I'd expected to speak with each trooper. I'd expected to probe for the *early* signs of this disease. (Stiff neck and rash were later developments.) I'd expected to ask, for example, about symptoms of fever and headache, for aches and chills, or nausea or sensitivity to light. To catch spinal meningitis early you had to be alert for flu-like symptoms. This exam was all about signs, not symptoms; about what I saw, not what they felt. And about seeing many troopers in a very short period of time. That lieutenant saved all our bacon, his men from a delayed assessment, me from embarrassment.

Naturally, I was uncomfortable with this military way but, really, how much of my discomfort was due to the unceremonious abortion of my authority as a doctor, a *captain*-doctor? And how much due to my personal associations? As a child, during the World War II years, I'd been hospitalized, myself, with meningitis, complicated by encephalitis. My father was away at war. I'd had spinal taps. I remember the nurses trying to cheer me by telling me to imagine the intravenous pole as my private "Christmas tree." (They'd decorated it.) But my family didn't celebrate Christmas, and I didn't feel safe enough to tell them. I felt so alone. I remember becoming delirious and hallucinating and asking my mother, during a visit, why little men were climbing on her chair. (The little men didn't frighten me. They intrigued me. What were they up to?) But I do remembered missing the comfort and reassurance that comes with something familiar, things the way they were supposed to be, and where everyone got to say how they felt.

There were no further cases of spinal meningitis while I was at Fort Bliss. The threat of the disease dissipated and, with that, periods of quiet and relaxation returned to this extended period of my waiting before deployment to Vietnam. I didn't feel quiet and relaxed, however. I felt a strange disquiet from the inactivity. I called it boredom, and considered my time wasted. I decided I was cynical and found petty annoyances to complain about. But I did learn a few things about myself from this down time, like my limits and my "buttons." I learned, too, that having a break with lots of time on one's hands isn't all it's cracked up to be. This is especially the case when there's lots going on in your head that you're trying not think about.

A Soldier's Friends: Joking, Griping, Bravado and the Illusion of Empowerment

There was, always looming, the reality of war, violence, and danger. Ironically, there were false friends available that proved to be a soldier's true friends. The joking, griping, bravado — what civilians would call denial — all effectively contributed to our being able to not think the unthinkable, to tolerate the intolerable, and to control ourselves (while, paradoxically, preserving and protecting our reality-testing) through the illusion of empowerment. If you could convert a documentary, as it were, into a farce and then give it a name and spit it out and laugh at it, you were in control. You had the last word (or could pretend to). You weren't so easily distracted by the gravitas of what something was really about. I remember during one exercise focusing on the caption I'd have put to the image of my facing a gas-chamber exercise. After being instructed in the proper wearing of a gas mask we lined up before a very large and long tent. I stood to the side to watch the men come out the other end without helmet and without mask looking ill and out of it. And when I finally went in, the last one in, I found myself facing 16 funny-looking guys wearing gas masks standing around a smoking pot in the center of the tent. My collar was up, tissue tucked around my neck, and my hands dug deep into my pockets. As I stood at attention and listened to the instructor — I was to remove my mask and state my name and serial number, then leave — these captions came to mind: "Oh, go on, Beanie. Take a puff." And: "Bill. Did you do it? No? Tom, did you do it? No? Bernard...." When you are joking, like griping, you experience a comfortable edge of superiority, an edge that can at least keep you from thinking about being just another pawn on somebody else's game board, which I was; we all were. At least, that.

One Chronic, Virulent, Treatment-Resistance Infection: Anti-Semitism

I had the opportunity to join a group in our training company relaxing in the mess, talking over coffee. The debate was whether President Truman "saved Western Europe" while his successor, Ike Eisenhower, "did nothing," or whether President Truman — called by one doctor, "Harry Asshole" — lost Asia in World War II and his predecessor, FDR, was a "criminal." I kept out because I understood little of politics. The only opinion I voiced was that President Truman had guts and principle because he lifted the arms embargo to Palestine in 1948. From there, the discussion took a sharp turn. The "Harry Asshole" voice in the group made a pointed reference to the "Christian" West.

Other voices immediately corrected this; "You mean, *Judeo*-Christian West." But "Harry Asshole" held his ground. "There's nothing Judeo about our West," he insisted. I made the obvious correction here and he retorted, "Jews never made the transition." As we digested this he completed that thought: "They were left behind."

"Made what transition?" I asked, feigning ignorance but knowing full well not only what he meant and where this was going but also where it was coming from. When he went on to speak of the love Christianity brought to civilization I reminded him of the abuse of Jews that regularly accompanied that "love."

"Every time I have a discussion with a group of guys," he now griped, "the topic of anti–Semitism always comes up and it's always the Jew that brings it up." Someone in the group corrected him, "*You* brought up the anti–Semitism." He seamlessly countered with, "Jews are responsible for anti–Semitism. They're always thinking about it. They always bring the subject up."

I had just spent part of the last two days in synagogue attending High Holiday services where prayers were said in the memory of the millions of Jews murdered in the war simply for being Jews, and that was in our own life-time. I told him it was wrong not to remember. He disagreed. "That was years go," he declared, "and it's best forgotten; it's all over." Another voice joined in. "That's not true. It can happen again at any time and anyplace. People haven't changed." And another voice (it was Yario, from Chicago). "With a truck and a day I could ride Chicago's streets and gather a pretty good facsimile of the old-time Brown Shirts. Jews don't create anti–Semitism." Yario continued: "Why did the Ecumenical Council spend so much time debating the issue of deleting the Christ-Killer bit?" He was referring here to the ongoing Catholic Church deliberations on this theme, roused no doubt by some painful introspection. (The church deliberations would conclude later that month in a document, "Nostra Aetate." Vatican II would go on record as officially condemning anti–Semitism, the hatred of Jews.)

And just when we thought this detour of our discussion group was over, my "Harry Asshole" friend managed to have the last word, a final rejoinder. "Another thing I don't like about Jews," he concluded: "They study and study. In any group it's always the Jews who get the best marks."

So, here we were, training to become champions in the battle to contain one virulent infection while, in our midst, we had to deal with a carrier of another. Ironic. A captain in the United States Army. A doctor. Not only a doctor but someone whose military medical occupation specialty (MOS) was D3005, preventive medicine. And he didn't even see he was spreading a sickness. Couldn't even see he was infected. Communism wasn't going to be the only potentially lethal infection out there needing containment.

Those situations in which I encountered anti–Semitism were always awkward, my response so lame. Following the infection model, ought I have focused on treatment and eradication? Ought I have focused on containment with an eye to preventing its spread? Or, ought I have concentrated on the anger, frustration, and helplessness I would always feel inside myself? Silence was never an option but, too often, happened by default. It was impossible to know the "right" response, even in hindsight; at least a response that would make *me* feel better. In my case I couldn't (and still can't) get beyond: "You piece of SHIT. You're a disgrace to the uniform and our profession." The good news was there would be other opportunities. Unfortunately, that was also the bad news.

3

I Volunteer for a
Special Program

Caregiving as Counter-Insurgency — MILPHAP

In my initial months in basic training, solicitations were periodically made for volunteers for programs that were short of doctors, such as the Special Forces, the 101st Airborne, and one stateside research facility inside a military base that came with the stipulation that you accept Top Secret clearance, never publish your research, never speak of it, either, and likely work with foreign personnel.

One caught my attention. It was a U.S. State Department program. It involved being on loan, as it were, to the Vietnamese Ministry of Health and taking the place of the Vietnamese civilian doctors now away doing military service. It entailed practicing general medicine among civilians. It was classified as counter-insurgency because it would recover the trust and allegiance of the people to their government. My hand shot up. They took my name. Optimal military readiness of American GIs would no longer be my prime directive. A Vietnamese civilian's well-being would. This felt right.

The program was called "Military Provincial Hospital Augmentation Program," and I was accepted. My orders were changed. There would be MILPHAP teams composed of three physicians, one medical administrative officer, and 12 enlisted technicians. Each team would be assigned to a specific provincial hospital where it would work under the supervision of that province's chief of medicine. From that base of operations the team would make mobile trips to the district infirmary or dispensaries and smaller installations down to the hamlet-level aid stations to augment their depleted staff. I would be part of the first wave of six teams to go over. (By the end of 1970, teams from the army, navy, and air force would be on the ground in 25 of South Vietnam's 44 provinces.) MILPHAP was set up to be sophisticated, far-reaching, military, and permanent, a major objective being the improvement of the medical skills of the Vietnamese. Supplies would come through Ministry of Health channels, not U.S. Army supply channels. Meanwhile, on stand-by, I was scheduled for additional training.

We were all on a learning curve. It was very much a work in progress. (Even the name would go through several iterations before being finalized. Role-playing yesterday's drama was an obvious example of playing catch-up. One exercise at Camp Bullis was called Survival, Evasion, and Escape, the focus being on evading an enemy who wanted to catch us even though anyone reading a newspaper could see that ours was an enemy proficient enough in hiding that nobody seemed able to find them. (Perhaps a more relevant focus might have been how to connect meaningfully with skeptical allies with a track record of foot-dragging.) Another exercise postulated a hypothetical enemy incursion into America. But anyone watching the news on the television knew that our enemy in Vietnam wasn't interested in seizing land but rather in capturing the allegiance, or neutrality, of the people who supplied them with food, information, and recruits. Then there was the image of a rescue operation by Number One Americans (like me) although anyone coming back could tell you that, parallel to the Vietnamese Public Health System, there was an indigenous (or "Chinese") healthcare system that was respected, easy to understand, and affordable, and surely with a consequence for any foreigner disrespecting that local, traditional "practitioner."

I didn't cut them slack, because I knew something was missing even though I couldn't put my finger on it. I had so many questions. How does one prepare for a civic action mission that would be centered on providing public health services — Western medicine — to Asian civilians during wartime and in a place where every zone is a war zone? How does one prepare for a mission whose ultimate purpose is getting civilians who have been repressed and abused for years by a distant, disinterested, and tyrannical government to trust their leaders again or, at least, remain indifferent to the Vietcong petitions or demands? How does one collaborate on time-driven projects when perceptions of time differ, where traditions of patience with tolerance are certain to clash with traditions of impatience with action? How does one prepare to be a helpful American in a country where direct eye contact can feel aggressive, a firm handshake threatening, and a pointed finger disrespectful? And where anyone you deal with or care for may be the enemy after sundown? More to the point, how does one prepare for the inevitable personalities, politics, customs, systems, and corruptions, now waiting, like elephants in the room, to blindside us once we got there? (And I'm speaking of both theirs and ours.)

The Elephants in the Room

No one mentioned to us the fact that the enemy insurgency in South Vietnam was not only strong but getting stronger. Or noted the years that American advisors had been arguing for reforms that had been steadfastly resisted by the Diem government of South Vietnam. No one explained that this new idea of not just rooting out insurgents but also turning the common people against them was critical because time was so short. Any land reforms, for example, offered at this point would likely be too few, if not too late altogether. Providing Western healthcare was envisioned as a way to inspire people to withhold their support from the increasingly brutal, revenge-minded Vietcong, who didn't hesitate to kill those who withheld from them. In a sense, the subtext of my narrative is my encounter with those same elephants that drove those former advisors to distraction and that, during my tour, repeatedly moved to crush me and keep me and my team from doing our job.

But those clashes weren't why, in my view, our mission failed. In my view it failed because of a flaw in its design, a design that joined a military objective to a humanitarian mission and would have military orders clashing with a doctor's Hippocratic Oath while providing no tools, lights, or map out of that ethical thicket for the hapless doctor. The irony was that the hearts and minds — the affection and support — that mattered most over the long haul turned out to be American, not Vietnamese. It would be American affection and our support for our American government, not that of the Vietnamese for theirs, that ultimately made the difference. (America wasn't beaten in this war, just outlasted. The support of the American people simply petered out.)

Meanwhile, what do you do, or who might you turn to, about obligatory formalities prior to getting down to business, mindful that an error might lead to your being shunned? Here's an example. You are invited to lunch by a Vietnamese. You don't know if it is a friendship gesture or more, a special honor — something offered to thank you — or a ruse. Who is he, anyway? Do you make sure you have a good appetite so you eat everything that is offered? Or do you snack first so as not to eat too much, not appear greedy? Or should you leave food, or offer food to others who might be there? Or not eat any food until it's checked out? Do you offer a blessing? Wait for a blessing? What do you do? Do you bring your weapon? Decline the invitation? I wanted to discuss this sort of thing. (This was an actual situation I faced in Vietnam.)

I'll note here, as a caveat, that I was never aware of this civic action program serving as cover for any covert military special operation. The Vietcong's aim to kidnap MILPHAP doctors, once this program was underway, arose not from motives of retaliating, punishing, or ransom, but rather for securing our medical services for their people.

We Become the 734th Medical Detachment, MACV Advisory Team 33

We would be three doctors, two captains, and a major who'd be the commander of the team. Since there was a shortage of majors the oldest doctor would be our commander. Stanley F. Banach, from Allentown, Pennsylvania, became commander of our team, the 734th Medical Detachment, MACV Advisory Team 33. I was second in command, the executive officer. William Baxley from Macon, Georgia, was our surgeon. Our administrative officer was Lieutenant Henry Brown from Columbia, South Carolina, career Army.

The twelve enlisted men, according to the book, would include a sergeant, four dispensary specialists, four dispensary assistants, one medical lab specialist, one clerk typist, and one medical assistant. These twelve would have primary training in either x-ray, pharmacy, and laboratory work and would be cross-trained in a second. (Unlike the army, the navy and air force had their men in the service for three years, all field trained in their specialties at the time of deployment.) Our team included Staff Sgt. E6 Lehman E. Strickland from Abington, Alabama; Clarence Prevo, Sp. 5 E5 from Pensicola, Florida; Sterling O. Sanders, Sp. 5 E5 from Washington, D.C.; Ellsworth N. Halvorson, Sp. 4 E4 from Tacoma, Washington; Leslie B. Maxwell, Jr., Sp. 4 E4 from Detroit, Michigan; Wilbert L. Davis, Jr., Pfc. E3 from Brooklyn, New York; Leon Harris, Pfc. E3 from Chicago, Illinois; Robert Aragon, Pfc. E2 from Albuquerque, New Mexico; Ted E. Davidson, Jr., Pfc. E2 from Dallas, Texas; John E. Guingrich, Pfc. E2 from Sparland, Illinois; Daniel G. Melberg, Pfc. E2 from Anoka, Minnesota; and Alfonso Rodriguez, Pfc. E2 from Salinas, California.[1]

Portents were not auspicious. Our pedigree, for one thing, was notably overrated and unheroic. Some of our men were neither volunteers nor field trained in dual specialties as advertised. Melberg recalls:

> After high-school I started going to the University of Minnesota college of liberal arts. About 2 months into my first semester I got a notice from my draft board to report for a physical. While I was in the post office building waiting for the bus someone came out of the office, called my name, and told me my student deferment had come through. By then I had already withdrawn from school and made preparations for becoming a soldier. So I went to the recruiting office and enlisted. Being young and stupid I enlisted for Airborne. Luckily, my eyesight wasn't good enough so I found my way into the Medical Corps and laboratory training. When I graduated I was assigned to MILPHAP [Pvt. E2 Daniel Melberg, personal communication].

Rodriguez adds:

> When we were chosen as medics it was scary because the only thing I knew of medicine was from having been in the Future Farmers of America in

high school and having been a hog farmer. I knew animal husbandry and how to castrate. I had also been cross-trained in dentistry and generators [Pvt. E2 Alfonso Rodriguez, personal communication].

As for me, it turns out I wasn't even supposed to be on this team any more. I was to be transfered to the 73rd Medical Detachment to be their major and company commander. Jim Whittenberg, the 73rd's current CO, was to deploy as a replacement for the 19th, already in place, because one of the doctors on that team had recently been ejected for insubordination. Meanwhile, a Captain Branch was to be my replacement. (Thankfully, I was allowed to remain where I was.) As for our mission — especially our destination and time of departure — these were classified as secret, our orders euphemistically referring to our destination as a "restricted area overseas." The colonel who'd trained the first group to go over had meanwhile become so proud of what he'd accomplished that he not only published a detailed article about their activities in the base newspaper and arranged press and TV coverage for their send-off, he pasted a large map of Vietnam on his office walls with pins locating his people. (He was court-martialed.) Then the news reached us that one MILPHAP team that deployed ahead of us was now sitting in Saigon and no one knew what to do with them. It seems the Vietnamese chief of medicine at their assigned provincial hospital didn't want them. To compound our vague sense of a SNAFU (now approaching TARFU and FUBAR status), rumor had it that Army General (Doctor) James William Humphreys, who'd been assigned the task of caring for us, didn't believe in the MILPHAP mission in the first place. To add injury to insult, just prior to our departure, one of our sergeants was mugged in town and hospitalized with lacerations and rib fractures. (He still deployed with us.) Even the weather, the humidity reaching 93 percent, seemed against us.

Is there any wonder I dreamed the following dream when it came time to deploy? In the dream I am watching a number of planes disgorge paratroopers far in the distance. Suddenly, amid the billowing white silk chutes comes a figure, spread-eagled and cartwheeling as he falls through the figures in the air toward the ground. They are all Vietnamese. I find myself sitting in a Piper Cub, flying along, preparing to drop a man who was going to be a coast-watcher. The pilot says he'll drop him at four feet. The plane skims along at very slow speed at grass level, then climbs. Once in the clouds the engine shuts off. We fall straight down with our tail dipped low. Then the engine comes on and we climb again. Later I am falling like a bullet, in a plane, towards the ground to crash. I know I am only watching a movie recovered from a plane that had crashed, but there isn't a screen for this movie. I see the view through the side panel windows. I am apprehensive but also reassured that it is only a film. Then I am standing in a place that is not unlike the laundry room of my childhood home. My mother is there. People are speaking about parachute jumping and I comment, "I made two parachute jumps." Then my mother becomes angry and hysterical.

My Talisman

In a moment of nostalgic bravado, I took from home during my final leave a navy knife my father had given me years before. My father's ship, the attack transport, USS *Barnett* APA-5, formerly an English passenger steamer but bought and converted for war by the U.S. Navy, saw action in all three theaters of World War II, the Atlantic, the Mediterranean, and the Pacific. It was there at Guadalcanal, Italy, Normandy and Okinawa, and it made it home safely. While that war was raging I had opportunity, as a small child, to board the *Barnett*. It had come to Newport News, Virginia, for dry dock repairs, and that was the opportunity for a family reunion. My mom bundled my brother, sister, and me aboard a train and we went down to Newport News and stayed in a one of scores of Quonset huts[2] on base during a part of the *Barnett*'s month in dry dock. I was six or seven years old. My dad gave me the navy knife then. It was in my mom's safe-keeping, locked up in my dad's study until he returned home for keeps in 1949. But, still, throughout my childhood and adolescence, I don't remember touching it or holding or carrying it. (I must have; I was a boy.) At any rate I knew where it was but I had no use for it until it was time to go overseas.

That navy knife represented something to me. Good luck? My father? Me? Our manliness? Our connection? Probably all of them. I never gave that question any thought, though. I never wondered. Probably because I didn't care to know the answer. Not back then, anyway. As to why a talisman at all, I'm a grandfather now and the answer to that is now obvious. I was going on a trip. It was my "snuggle."

4

In-Country: Saigon
(Ho Chi Minh City)

At 1730 hours (5:30 p.m.) Tuesday, June 21, 1966, after a 26-hour flight that began at Kelly Air Base in San Antonio and made fueling stops at Travis Air Field in San Francisco and Wake Island, flying at 500 mph at 35,000 feet in a crowded and cramped two-window C-141 cargo plane of the Military Airlift Command that carried all our baggage, sitting alongside doctors packed like sardines along rows of canvas jump seats (parachuter seats) with no room to move about, I arrived at Tan Son Nhat Airport outside of Saigon. Because we'd crossed the international date line we actually gained a day. We'd departed San Antonio at 0030 hours (12:30 a.m.) Monday.

98 percent personnel going to VN travel in 707s. We're the 2 percent who travel on cargo planes. To go to the john you had to climb over the baggage and, even there, you had to crawl over GI's trying hard to stretch out to sleep. It was hell.

First Test — Making a Medical Diagnosis: I Fail

Almost immediately there was this unforgettable and humbling moment. While we stood, gathered in the MACV compound in Saigon (Ho Chi Minh City) — a group that included 18 physicians just off the plane from the States — one of the doctors felt ill. He became queasy and faint. Among the cluster of us doctors, myself included, who stepped in to try and help him, we must have asked him over and over about prior episodes like this, about gastrointestinal problems and cardiovascular problems. About anxiety attacks. We touched all the bases and everything was negative. The doctor in distress did his best, but there was nothing we could put a finger on that would show us

37

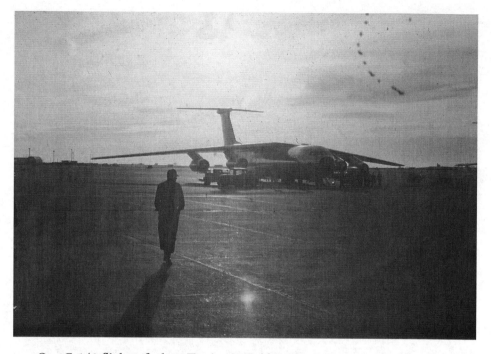

Our C-141 flight refuels at Travis Air Field in San Francisco, Monday, June 20, 1966.

what to do. The irony here was lost in the competition among us doctors trying to be the one to make the right diagnosis. The irony was that our predicament and this momentary embarrassment was possibly a portent of what lay ahead for us, namely that we might not be up to *that* job, either. It turned out it was only ordinary dehydration from the long flight. Some swallows of water brought relief. Ordinary hydration. We were that wound-up. Maybe that dehydrated ourselves.

We spent our first night in the MACV Headquarters compound in the heart of the city. It's an old, French hotel with European elevators, tiny lobby, balcony to each room, and a courtyard. All buildings like this one have military police behind sandbags. Lots of construction. GI's sitting on sidewalks with kids, fixing their bikes or just talking. It's not pretty, at least where our bus drove. It was crowded with dirty alleys. Its hot and humid with intermittent downpours. The city is overcrowded, filthy and smelly, with tiny, skinny people in cone hats and pajamas hurrying along garbage-lined streets.

Charlie [the Vietcong] knows about MILPHAP but he leaves us alone. Teams here since the fall have even gotten referrals from V.C. doctors!

Second Test — Facing the Camera: I Flee

Shortly after our arrival a Vietnamese TV crew approached our team. While I was the tallest and most conspicuous, Stan Banach, our CO, thankfully didn't hesitate to step forward and allow them to interview him. I was close enough to hear their first question: what were your first impressions of Vietnam? He spoke tactfully of how it reminded him of home. I moved away and never heard the rest of that interview, but I became aware of how unprepared I'd have been, how uncomfortable and on-the-spot I'd have felt. I'd surely have mangled that interview and that opportunity and certainly would have exposed the weak underbelly of the Mighty American Military Machine, namely, people like me who, while we don't hesitate to buy into that image ourselves when it suits our purpose, are poor candidates to represent it to the world in ad lib and uncensored moments like this.

I can remember to this day the kaleidoscope of sensory impressions and reactions that flooded me those first days in Vietnam, none of them easy to process let alone articulate. I remember, too, the tension of that moment when the TV crew approached us, between my wanting to please Vietnamese TV viewers (and my superiors) and be approved by them — we had no term such as "politically correct," back then — while, at the same time, wanting to be honest and speak the truth. And what was the truth? The truth was I was sore and tired. I was relieved and excited. I was nervous and apprehensive. And I was shamelessly hiding my misgivings, doubts, and insecurities — even from myself— behind that shield of my being an American and, as such, Number One. What's to worry about? I'm cool. We're cool. (*That* shield.)

These were the impressions I'd have gagged on: hot, sprawling, overcrowded, filth, pollution, and small, dirty cars —fleets of tiny Renault taxis — noisy motorbikes and scooters. Horse drawn carts. Small people wearing sandals or barefoot. People everywhere. Cone hats everywhere. Commotion. No obesity, no beards. Beautiful women with delicate features but bodies like nine year-olds. Naked children. Men wearing shorts. No couples walking together, let alone holding hands. Men walking together *and* holding hands. No tall buildings. Garbage lining the walks. People urinating against the walls, defecating alongside the curb. Uncomfortably humid. (It did *not* remind me of home.)

I was shallow and critical in such observations, inclined to see signs of a people overwhelmed and overtaken, needy and surely grateful for help, our help. I was inclined to forget what I had only recently read and learned, that these were people who had experienced more than 25 years of continuous war, meaning I was not ready to cut them the slack they'd earned, to step back and recognize that all the things I saw were signs of resilience and determination, fortitude and the ability to keep going in the worst of times.

Sometimes, you just know in your gut, prior to any thoughts registering in your awareness, that it's time to flee. This was one of them. I fled from the cameras.

MACV Orientation

Our first four days in Saigon we, the six MILPHAP Teams, stayed at the French hotel, Hotel Koepler, which had been leased from the Vietnamese by MACV. Here we received our canvas and leather jungle boots with removable metal insoles to stop punji stakes puncturing through, and jungle fatigues, etc. We had daily briefings. Briefings ranged from MACV history and organization to security, RVN air and naval operations to counterinsurgency operations, from what food to eat to not running to look out the window when you hear shooting, to which of the Vietcong Military Regions we'd be assigned to (from captured documents), to Rogers Rangers Standing Orders (1759). These included: No. 1, "Don't forget nothing," No. 15, "Don't sleep beyond dawn — dawn's when the French and Indians attack," and No. 19, "Let the enemy come till he's almost close enough to touch. Then let him have it and jump out and finish him up with your hatchet." The point: be mindful and alert. We learned the best brand of condom.

Hotel Koepler is a European style hotel located down a courtyard from the street, white stucco, and about 6 floors high with a balcony outside each room. A shuttered door opens onto the balcony. Our room is small with 3 double-decker beds. The john has a sink, toilet, and overhead shower spigot. So you shower (if the water is running) right there, even on the pot if you like doing the two things at once. The area is walled in with a sandbagged guard station outside by the gate. An MP and a VN policeman stand guard. I've taken some pictures but they tell me the shops won't develop these. Charlie uses photo shops to get his pictures of GI installations — the ground plan, defense systems, etc.

The Minister of Health welcomed us, General Humphrey said his piece, the MPs scared us. The United States Agency for International Development (USAID) confused us. There was no talk of mobs or demonstrations while we were there. The primary concern was terrorist bombing.

This is the text of the speech by the Vietnamese minister of health at that welcoming ceremony of the six incoming MILPHAP Teams (June 25, 1966):

Ladies and Gentlemen,
Once again I have the honor to be here with you to welcome the six MILPHAP Teams, one of the important health programs of our friendly

country, the United States of America, coming to Vietnam to assist our health activities.

Because of the war needs, we don't have enough health experts to care for the increasing number of wounded and sick patients, the Ministry of Health has to call for help from the nations of the Free World. Sympathizing with the sufferance of the Vietnamese people in this period of time, the United States has actively provided tremendous aids to Vietnam not only in military but also in other vital fields — economic, cultural, social, health. As for health, under the health augmentation program, 12 MILPHAP Teams had [sic] arrived Saigon and are now assisting the provincial health services to provide medi-care and disease prevention to the people. By good-will, skillful techniques, and hard work, the experts of the MILPHAP Teams have gained deep affection of Vietnamese people in all classes. This helps to fade away some misunderstandings, if it is so, between the two nations in order to fight side-by-side for the democracy and freedom.

Today, on behalf of the government and the people of Vietnam, I sincerely appreciate those of you in the MILPHAP Teams who don't mind the danger, the difficulty to come here to share with us the responsibility of development and improvement of health in Vietnam, contributing to the ultimate victory of all people. I would like to send you my warmest welcome, wish you the best of luck, and success in your mission.

Thank you.

I reassured my family back home:

Assure everybody that things are going well for me. Saigon seems quiet now. We're well-guarded. I'm in good health, rested, and showered. Had a good BM (considering that trip plus the diarrhea-causing chloroquine anti-malarial pill — I guess they cancelled each other out) this morning. There is potable water here and a snack bar in this compound.

Children are fascinated by body hair. They walk up to me with their shoeshine boxes, "OK, Number 1, shine Joe, OK" and I'll say, no. Then they'll stand there pulling the hair on my arms.

I bought souvenirs at a Saigon market including an unusual chess set. The king was a tall, bearded, Confucius-like figure, the bishop not unlike a Buddha, the castle a pagoda, and pawns busts of oriental figures with cone hats. Since I had, back home, an equally unusual chess set with medieval figures of knights, bishops, castles, etc. I thought, once home, I'd set up and display one against the other. (I never did. Back home I no longer found that image amusing.)

Our MILPHAP Team was oriented to some interesting dos and don'ts that became, for me, like a window on the nature of the insurgency warfare I'd been reading about. We were directed not to stand in groups, for example.

While shopping, only one person shops at a time while the other is lookout. When getting in a cab and closing the door, quickly make sure it opens again. Never enter or exit a cab within 25 yards of a military police station.

On the 4th day we moved to the Chinese quarter of Saigon, Cholon, and into the Hotel Coliseum.

> *Sandbags and oil drums in front and one MP on guard. Windows are taped to prevent flying glass. They were hit a week before we got there. A V.C. agent tossed a grenade at some GIs at the bus stop and then set off a Claymore mine to cover his retreat. 13 wounded, none dead. I spoke to a Korean officer who just came out of the hospital. He said he saw a smoking box tossed at him "and they all ran." His comment. "Vietnamese Police Number 10." (Everything here is rated No. 1 or No. 10.)*
>
> *There were guards at the first 3 landings (the staircase is an outside staircase) with clubs. I was lucky to be on the 5th floor with an excellent view of the city and the flares over the river at night (balconies and patios outside rooms like in Paris). We were 10 in the room but we had electricity which would sometimes be shut off and we'd sit by candlelight. Overhead fans and toilet-showers with water usually running. Drinking water set each day on the tables in old gin and whiskey bottles. Artillery thumping every night as part of the harassment of V.C. along the river.*

"Separateness" and "Nicknaming": Two Flies in Our Ointment

Being physically safe was a priority in Saigon. I was relieved and happy to be put up at these old French hotels with military police as guards. But, in my relief, it never occurred to me how much this separateness might, at some point, be a spoiler to a mission such as ours. Being billeted like this with other Americans in well-guarded French hotels that set us apart and kept us from (and cautious about) contact with Vietnamese civilians surely registered with these people as well as constricting our own personal comfort zones. How could this inspire feelings of affection, let alone connection or trust? If I were on the other end of this I'd be dutifully impressed and intimidated, to be sure, and more than a little envious, but mainly I'd feel put off. I don't like having my losses and limitations, my neediness and vulnerability, shoved in my face. I saw this separateness as a fly in our ointment, in the humanitarian balm we had come to apply to our ally's wounds.

I was more than happy to continue to have access to typewriters to record my observations, to find stories in the myriad of experiences I was having. It is obvious now — it wasn't back then — how much my writing served to take a complex and disquieting experience and render it comprehensible to myself, not just interesting to someone with whom I'd share it. Writing does that for a writer. It tames and calms your nerves when you are unable to find the right words to process a cluster of emotions. But — and this is my point — how was this different from the men I'd been encountering and who'd been in Vietnam a long time, using words for a similar purpose but in a distinctively offensive, destructive way? I'm referring to GIs speaking about Vietnamese as "Slopes" (from the slope or slant of the eyes from the epicanthic folds) and the Rhade (E' De), Mnung, Jarai (Gia Rai), and Koho (K'Ho) tribesmen all as "Yards" (from the word *Montagnard*). When we objectify the other with a label don't we diminish them? Don't we dismiss and control them; if not the "them" in reality then the "them" in our minds? Over time and usage, don't "they" become for us not just "other," but Other, in the same way alien becomes Alien? In short, were we not ensuring our emotional well-being through the expedient of disrespect, of labeling, of name-calling? I was. This was the other fly in our healing ointment.

If the heart of an advisory relationship resides in the relationship itself, then these two flies in our ointment were potential corrupters, corrupters of our mission through corrupting us. Looking back it seems obvious how this naming and separateness, insidiously and effectively, can almost take back whatever it is we think we're offering and delivering. Or take back whatever it is someone thinks they have already taken away from us. I'm thinking of China replacing the name, Peking (our name) with Beijing and insisting others do the same. And India, likewise, replacing Bombay (our name) with Mumbai. Burma and Myanmar. And Kenya shedding the soul-crushing name their colonizers gave them, British East Africa.

Back in 1966 in Vietnam I understood none of this. I felt the seductive pull to use those labels, "Slopes" and "Yards" — I could feel its bonding effect on the "us" versus the "them" — but it offended and scared me. Its bravado advertised insecurity. Also, it was unfair. If our enemy, the Vietcong or V.C., were worthy of the respectful appellation, "Charlie" or "Victor Charlie" (from the NATO phonetic alphabet), why not our allies as well? Worse, in informal conversations (and even those without alcohol) terms such as "Slopes" and "Yards," became regularly interchangeable with "mother-fuckers" (spoken almost affectionately as a familiar tag). But it made me sick and poses this necessary question: When an officer hears enlisted men in his command employing these labels to facilitate team-bonding, ought he or she intervene? (Keep in mind that, if our team was any example, enlisted men are a diverse group that includes professional soldiers and citizen-soldiers; pro-war, anti-war, and conscientious objectors; white, black, and Latino; Christians and Jews;

Northerners and Southerners and urban and rural guys; not just officers and enlisted men. Keep in mind, too, that, if ours was any example, teams were not natural fits in terms of friendship and leadership. And also keep in mind that team morale can make the difference in the success of a mission.) So, ought that officer intervene? Scold? Give a harmless talk about respect and civility? To my knowledge, this was never an issue for our MILPHAP Team. I doubt it was an issue for any MILPHAP Team.

Meanwhile, back at the ranch (literally), President Lyndon Johnson, a Texan with a southern drawl, famously, unabashedly, and always, mispronounced "Vietnam" as "Veet-nahm." He never, to my knowledge, made the slightest effort towards the correct pronunciation, "Vee-Yet-Nam." "Veet-naam," Johnson's version translates to, "Sick Duck." So, GI slang that disrespects had a respectable bloodline.

Connections and Misfires

A V.C. suspect was stopped along our route from the Ministry of Health with a grenade attached to his bicycle.

Got a discount in cigarettes because I asked for them in Vietnamese.

We are advised to get MILPHAP Team emblems because we want Charlie to identify us. One of the men on our team designed an emblem for the 734th. Our CO ordered copies made.

Demolition team arrived at hotel after sundown. Someone thought he saw a Claymore mine. False alarm.

I had spent an evening in the street surrounded by kids who gave me Vietnamese language lessons. I had made notes in my notebook. As I turned to leave them I turned my cap sideways for a laugh. The same kids were out front next day. They ran over and smiled and turned their hats sideways and made writing motions. We reviewed my lessons.

The children are clever at pantomime and will repeat words till I get them right. I needed a light and one kid ran next door and gave me a book of matches and wouldn't take it back. Although their parents seem to take no interest or show authority over them they are friendly, generous, and without any trace of destructiveness.

One of my sergeants had terrible heat cramps. Didn't take his salt tablets.

Heavy downpours of monsoon rain. Comes frequently and lasts several hours, followed by damp, muggy heat.

The first part of the bus ride—Navy-scheduled bus routes (wire mesh over all windows as precautions against thrown grenades)—was from hotel through teeming, congested Chinese market, the bus rubbing sides against stalls; an unending mob in front of us, firecrackers (hell on our nerves) outside.

Women are beautiful to look at. Men appear to show no interest in them. The women and girls look at you, at your eyes.

Navy people get nasty and shout at the hotel girl when their laundry isn't ready. They slap the Vietnamese bus driver (saying, "Hey!") when he appears to be driving in circles. They smash the locker door in the hotel room because it won't open. They don't return salutes of my men.

An Air Force sergeant on the bus home complained about the bumpy ride and the lack of adequate street lights and, as we approached the Hotel Coliseum, said, "They ought to bomb this place. I think I'll send a note to Charlie." He repeated this to the MP on guard duty who quietly said, "Don't say that. I'm out front."

I ran into the street when a Vietnamese kid's hat fell off as he bicycled past the Victoria Hotel. I handed it to him before I was aware of police whistles and guns leveled. I'll never do that again.

The MPs are front-line soldiers, if there is a "front line." And they're sick of bombings. Don't dare stop your car in front of a U.S. building or the MP will blast you. They call the MPs and their Vietnamese counterparts, "untouchables." Don't touch them. They have enough headache with V.C. If a drunk GI gets smart or raises a hand to these guys, they'll shoot sooner than talk.

I ate lunch alone at Hong Kong Hotel. No wonder the waitress didn't understand my Vietnamese. She speaks only Chinese. She teases and punches freely. She's 29 and looks 18. She sat down to go over my booklet on medical questions in Vietnamese, giving Chinese translation. Then she wrote me a note. It said, "I get off work at two o'clock."

5

The Central Highlands:
Initiation

Central Highlands, Vietnam

Seventy percent of South Vietnam, a country about the size of New England, is mountains and beautiful lakes with dense forests and thickets, rolling plains with head-high brush — "mountain jungle" — part of the vast network of mountain chains and high plateaus that link the countries of Indochina and stretches for more than 1,500 miles northwest to the Himalayas. While spacious, it was occupied by only 15 percent of the people of South Vietnam in 1966, people racially different from the ethnic Vietnamese, the so-called Montagnards. That's where I was going.

Finding Our Place:
We Begin Wearing Blue Berets with a Tassel in Back

At dawn we bussed out. Just before we left MPs discovered a 200 lb. plastic bomb in a car parked alongside the Brinx Hotel where we ate many times. We picked up our weapons at the Koepler and then to Ton Son Nhut Airport for a C-47 flight north to Dar Lac Province and its capitol, Ban Me Thuot.

We were given .30 carbines — the M2 rifle from WW II — and 3 clips of 30 rounds each. I asked for a .45 handgun.

Why did I ask for a .45 pistol? Because my imagined risk was not that my hospital would be under attack or that my MACV Team 33 compound

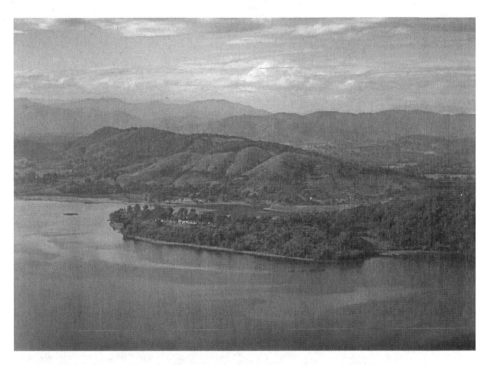

Lac Thien in Dar Lac province, today Dak Lak province (photograph from an L-19 reconnaissance aircraft).

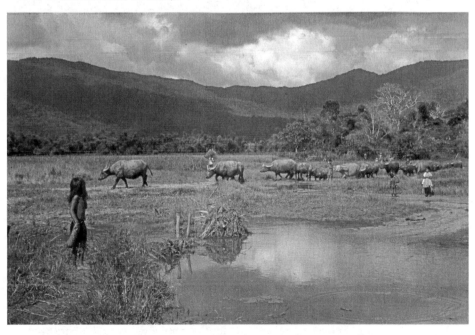

Lac Thien district, Dar Lac province, Central Highlands.

would be under attack. I'd seen the MACV security in Saigon; there'd be plenty of real soldiers around. It was that, on my trips into the countryside to visit district infirmary-dispensaries and hamlet aid stations, I'd be kidnapped. I wanted a weapon that would never be out of reach, even when both hands were occupied. Silly? Paranoid? Inappropriate? (They issued me the .45 pistol.)

Dar Lac (Darlac) covered the greater part of II Corps Area. Ban Me Thuot is its capital city. In South Vietnam, civilian administrative areas like province and district — think state and county — were partnered to military areas like corps, sector, and subsector. No, the two didn't always correspond and, no, the parallel lines of authority weren't always effectively managed. Dar Lac province is where the country bends like a comma around Cambodia. It was the traditional home to three Montagnard tribes, the Rhade, Koho, and Mnung, and was headquarters of the Vietnamese 23rd Division as well as home base for the Mennonite medical missionaries working at the Ban Me Thuot Leprosarium.

> From the air I could see that the people live in huts along tar-paved or red clay roads, with fences, chickens and pigs and cows everywhere. There is rich vegetation all over; flowers, flower trees, and tall grass, more rural village than mountain jungle.

We landed at the airport at Ban Me Thuot where we were welcomed by Michael Benge, USAID rural affairs provincial development officer, and Doctor Ton That Niem, director of Public Health region II, acting head of public health services of Dar Lac Province, medical director of the Dar Lac province hospital in Ban Me Thuot, and our team's immediate supervisor. A sister from the Benedictine convent was there to welcome us as well.

> We piled into Land Rovers for the 15 km ride into Ban Me Thuot. The sun was shining; it was pleasantly warm. We drove a tar-paved road through beautiful, rich land with neat and clean huts and farms, rubber plantations, corn fields, and clean, red clay yards. No Pepsi signs, no trash or garbage. Fences and sturdy huts, attractive, airy. Its monsoon season but the sun is out.

Our team would be directly responsible to Dr. Niem. USAID would finance operations. Security and room and board would be courtesy of MACV Advisory Team 33 Headquarters, which was the three-unit hunting lodge or chalet of former emperor Bao Dai for his guests, familiarly called "the Bungalow," and only a short walk from the lodge where the emperor himself stayed and from the province hospital. The MACV compound, which was surrounded by high concertina wire and flood-lit after dark, and where there were sandbagged defense positions beneath the elevated buildings, abutted the perimeter of a Special Forces "B" Camp. Enlisted men's quarters inside the compound were recently constructed barracks. The MILPHAP officers bunked with the other MACV officers, the advisors to the RVN division and the Regional/Popular Forces. (The Regional Force were mostly Rhade Montagnards, their officers being mainly ethnic Vietnamese from Saigon drafted for the duration. The Popular Force consisted of a hamlet's part-time soldiers. Their platoons were often older men, Rhade ex–French-colonial soldiers.) Like these MACV combat advisors we were allowed the option of wearing the blue beret with the tassel in back.

There are three identical A-Frame Swiss Chalet-style interconnected buildings with porch all around. Dark, mahogany-colored wood. They stand on firm pillars 12 feet off the ground. My room has a high ceiling with a double-decker and a single bed, bamboo cushion chairs, desk, bookcase, fan, screened door, and window. There is a bathroom separated by a curtain with drinkable tap water, huge tub, ice box. (Other MILPHAP teams got tents or huts. We've this!) My roommates are a captain and a lieutenant who are advisors for the RVN 23rd Division and the local Regional and Popular Forces, the "RF-PF"s.[1] Nice guys. They wear black berets. I'm drinking their beer now.

Just as there are instructions at the start of movies, flights, and voyages alerting people to emergency exits and procedures, the senior advisor for the 33rd Advisory Team, a colonel, held a practice alert shortly after we arrived. For the time being we doctors were assigned firing positions inside bunkers. I'd use the carbine they issued to me. Later, we'd be assigned to an aid station inside the compound. From time to time, there were practice alerts. (Sometimes they weren't practice.)

It means full battle gear and webbing. Stan tells me webbing is the shoulder straps to which you attach your "murder things." Everyone goes to an appointed defense position.

Our base of operations, the province hospital, located in the middle of this sprawling city of 50,000, traditional home to the Rhade people, joined recently by North Vietnamese refugees who'd fled Communism and were resettled here, was walking distance from the Bungalow. Rural Ban Me Thuot was close by. (I was told that the majority Montagnard population here were Catholic, inasmuch as French missionaries had considerable influence in these highlands.)

The city featured several wide boulevards lined by bougainvillea. After the rebellion that had erupted here in 1963, many of the fighters and leaders, under the banner of FULRO (a French acronym for United Front for Liberation of Oppressed Races), had retreated to Cambodia. Like our Vietnamese colleagues in healthcare and like the patients we'd be treating, we were a racially mixed bunch. Our radio call-name was Sport Grant.

*There is a center of town with crowded markets, shops — they sell stereo
and Hi-Fi equipment, bicycles, tailors, bookstores, food and, of course, lots
of junk. Here, as opposed to Saigon, the boulevards with huge trees lining
it are neat, clean, and picturesque.*

The spread-out provincial hospital had been largely turned over to the
Vietnamese military. A small portion, made up of elevated single-story stucco
structures and interconnecting pavilions (because of the monsoon rains) in
the French colonial style, remained as a civilian or public hospital. The two
sections of the hospital were separated by barriers. The civilian part included
a private or "pay" ward, a charity or "public" ward (with separate structures
for ethnic Vietnamese and Montagnards), a surgical suite and ward, a mid-
wife/obstetrical unit, an outpatient clinic with injection room, laboratory (for
urinalysis, blood chemistry, hematology, bacteriology, parasitology, and x-ray
services), pharmacy, and offices.

At the time MILPHAP arrived, the hospital was seriously and chronically
short of medicine and other supplies. In any case, no medications were dispensed on weekends. During times of severe shortage, patients picked up and
went home. One (female) civilian doctor and a visiting military surgeon were

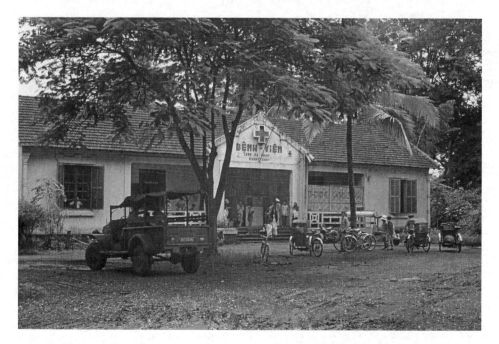

**Outpatient clinic entrance to the civilian section of Dar Lac province hospital.
Patients registered at the small booth at the top of the stairs.**

the only Vietnamese physicians overseeing all clinical care for civilians in the Province of Dar Lac. Two American military doctors, Capt. Wheeler of MACV Team 33 and Capt. Paulk of the 155th Aviation Company,[2] had been volunteering their time at the Montagnard charity ward. Capt. Banach and Sergeant Strickland were assigned to the "pay" ward, along with Pfcs. Robert Aragon, Alfonso Rodriguez, and Sp. 4 Ellsworth Halvorson. They would be working with a Vietnamese nurse and H Nhe, a Rhade nurse.

The doctor carries great weight, a tradition of the Mandarin system. The physician of old was wealthy, politically-oriented, and an important administrator. Their word for doctor is pronounced, "bok-see-ee." They're impressed when you tell them that's what you are.

Four bilingual youths, Duy (phonetically, "Z'wi"), Chinh, and the Nguyen brothers Hoan and Dinh (phonetically, "Din"), were our interpreters, employed by USAID. They'd been recommended to USAID by their high school English teacher, who'd asked them to apply. They scored highest on the application examination.

I'm healthy. No diarrhea or fever. A mosquito net hangs over my bunk. I shave daily even though a mustache seems a trademark among officers here. Our equipment hasn't yet arrived.

The customary military activities were our occasional mortaring around the outskirts of Ban Me Thuot or attempts to ambush convoys that left for Pleiku and Qui Nhon to the north and northeast. I went about in civilian clothes when the outpatient clinic was closed to emphasize the noncombatant nature of my presence and intentions. I neither carried nor needed a weapon.

I take a refreshing shower in the morning and have a good breakfast with eggs made to order. My clothes are cleaned and pressed when the house-boy brings them in and if there has been enough sunshine. We eat in the officer's mess, with salad, American dishes, iced tea (without the ice) served by Vietnamese girls. A houseboy cleans my room daily, polishes my boots, sews on insignias, sees the laundry gets done, and lowers the mosquito bed nets each afternoon.

I noticed and was intrigued by the differences between the Vietnamese of the lowland areas (the ethnic "Vietnamese") and those of the highlands, the so-called Montagnards. The latter had skin that was bronze (not yellow) and round eyes (not with the epicanthic fold, the "slant" eye), and they spoke atonal languages (not tonal or "sing-song"). I was troubled to learn that the traditional Vietnamese word for these Montagnard, *moi*, translates, roughly, to "savage." However, in recent years the term *moi* has been replaced by the

Vietnamese term that translates to "people of the plateau" or "Highlander." Phonetically, it sounds like "N'goo-we Tu-ung." (It reminded me of our own fairly recent language shift from "nigger" to "black.")

They are beginning to refer to these people as Highlanders to help include them in the Vietnamese community. These people are bronze skinned, tall, high cheek bones with long, straight black hair. Look at pictures of American Indians and you'll see a Highlander face. They appear mongoloid, as do American Indians, but no trace of the oriental (slant eyes, yellow skin, delicate features), if such is possible. Men wear pants and shirt or loin cloths. You see them walking to town with their spears and their women several steps behind. The women wear hand-woven ankle length skirts with beautiful maroon, yellow, orange, etc. embroidery along the hem and elsewhere. Babies are tied to their backs and baskets slung over their shoulders. They, too, nurse their babies in public and are bare-breasted on occasion. They speak a guttural dialect which the Vietnamese can't understand. Men and women both wear bracelets and ear-rings.

Capt. William Baxley and Pvt. Wilbert Davis were assigned surgical responsibilities, in support of the part-time Vietnamese military surgeon. Pfcs. John Guingrich and Dan Melberg were assigned to the laboratory. My

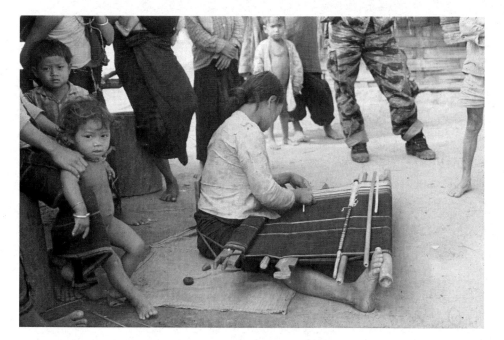

Montagnard (Mnung) weaver.

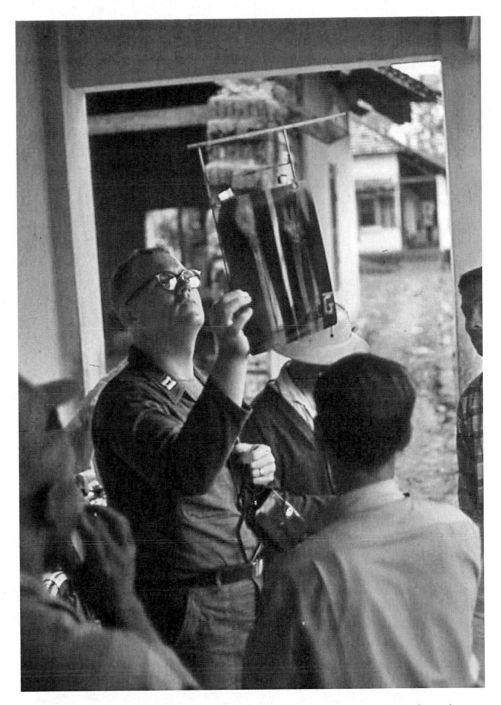

Capt. Baxley, our MILPHAP surgeon, stands outside the surgery ward on the porch where lighting is good and examines an x-ray. Note the partially destroyed structure behind him.

assignment, along with Sgt. Sanders and Pvt. Harris, was the outpatient clinic of the *benh-vien* (phonetically "bite-vien") or hospital. Lt. Brown shared an office with Dr. Niem's secretary, Co Hoa. For hospital staff meetings, Dr. Niem, who was fluent in English and French, and spoke Rhade, needed no interpreter. He repeated his Vietnamese comments first English and then Rhade.

> *The hospital people have been very friendly and courteous with us. Dr. Niem shakes hands with all of us when we depart. So far we've done the right things. For example, our first day visiting the hospital the RVN surgeon (who performs the only surgery on civilians) asked us to help him in an operation. Bill Baxley scrubbed in on the removal of a bladder stone of a Montagnard girl. Her father visited the girl in the recovery room and when Bill showed him the (larger than the largest marble) stone the man wept.*
>
> *When Stan and I entered the large, dilapidated shed — their storage house and only place large enough to hold all the staff — the people there stood up. As Dr. Niem introduced each of us they politely applauded and we then stood and bowed a little, embarrassed. While Dr. Niem was explaining our mission Bill came in. As he sat Dr. Niem introduced him and everyone smiled and clapped and Bill smiled back and nodded and said, "Thank you." When Stan was later asked for comments he said we'd all appreciate their teaching us any Vietnamese words they can during our work as we want to get to know the people and want them to get to know us. By the nods and smiles you could see he said the right thing.*

Our team was formally presented to the province chief, an RVN army colonel of II Corps. We sat in his very Western office while the monsoon rains poured down outside. Dr. Niem was there. We chatted about the weather. Also about the crops such as rubber, coffee, rice. We spoke about the hospital.

> *Then colonel slid back the wall-sized province map and rolled out another. He called it the Variola Map. Variola is the old name for smallpox. It was dotted with symbols of military units, regiments, battalions, — these were all V.C. Units. A platoon was here in Ban Me Thuot. He traced the highway running southwest to Saigon, Highway 2 running east to the coast, the road north to Pleiku, and then he held the curtain out of the way so we could see the Ho Chi Minh trail to our west. Not only does it pass us, a spur runs northeast of us whereby the V.C. supply the North Vietnam soldiers who have infiltrated here. Now I understand why the chart in Dr. Niem's office showing the personnel makeup of his infirmary-dispensaries in the districts of Dar Lac are all blank. That is why we'll probably never send out mobile teams. Three of four Dar Lac Districts are under Vietcong control.*

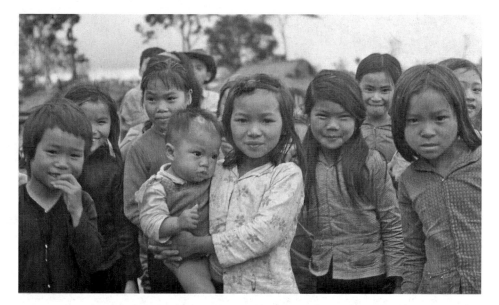

Children were conspicuously curious.

Ban Me Thuot was attractive, interesting, and safe enough. We walked alone and unarmed about town, through the market place, watched the people, and shopped. The people appeared comfortable with us, pleased we were there.

Social life in town is limited to a movie house, "lounges" with prostitutes, and sidewalk cafes that serve beer. The GIs go to the lounges when there is an armed guard in front or watch movies at the Bungalow. I sit and play chess and drink vermouth. During afternoon siesta when the hospital locks up and patients go home I play softball or volleyball with other officers. In front of the Bungalow is a large soccer field. We are 100 feet from the center of town, separated by barbed wire on one side. In the other direction you walk out into mountain jungle after half-mile.

Our mission was to augment the existing system, not reform it, and to assist our Vietnamese colleagues, not compete with them or, worse, show them up. To deliberately present yourself as Number One, in addition to it being arrogant, insulting, and inappropriate, would be contrary to orders.

It was necessary for us to know and keep in mind that our Vietnamese allies were tired of promises not kept and hopes dashed and had learned the hard way to be self-reliant where they could, to trust the familiar, even if only adequate. Even if barely adequate. To improvise. To bend rules if it put their families first. But I didn't yet know this. This I had yet to learn. (I didn't know that, either.)

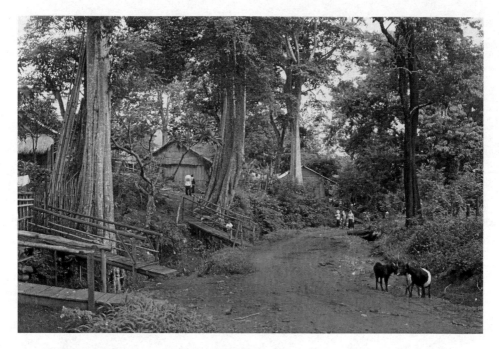

Rural Ban Me Thuot, unpaved and without litter, often hilly, was always scenic and inviting.

There is nothing now about my mission which is confidential. The rain has stopped and it's a clear, sunny day. The dark, wooden bungalows stand out against the background of trees and flowers. It's 2:00 P.M. and I'll go home for a nap.

That MILPHAP Team No One Knew What to Do With: A Follow-Up

That misplaced MILPHAP Team is being used to treat out-patients in various clinics in and around Saigon. We met Lou DiTullio and his interpreter who told us what it was like. They travel around in an open jeep with their carbines. They have no base hospital as we do. Their security is provided by some RF-PF'ers. We had to laugh at these "instant" soldiers. Lou described how he took them outside of town to the firing range for some familiarization firing. While they blasted away at the targets, V.C. on the far side were firing back at them. They didn't even realize this. Lou had to shoo his men away; they simply didn't know.

The Navy MILPHAP Team That Arrived with Us: A Follow-Up

In Bat (sp?) Lac Province where one of the Navy MILPHAP Teams that trained and came over here with us is stationed, there was a firefight several nights ago. Local RVN Rangers discovered that two V.C. units were fighting each other so they settled down and zapped everybody with artillery. From the prisoners they learned that the V.C. mission was to kidnap the MILPHAP Team. The MILPHAP Team wasn't where it was supposed to be, it was 10 miles out of the way. The V.C. inadvertently fired on each other. This blows our notion that MILPHAP is a good-conduct pass. We were all thankful that the Navy Team is OK. We aren't really concerned for our safety, though. Word is the American 4th Division is planning to set up quarters 10 miles from here. We have no intention of sending mobile teams out for a long, long time, if ever.

Montagnards vs. Ethnic Vietnamese

From the start, accounts were told to us by other Americans comparing and contrasting Montagnards with ethnic Vietnamese. It was like an informal part of our orientation to this assignment in the central highlands, and it wasn't simply about a rivalry between two allied military units operating in the area, the Civilian Irregular Defense Group or CIDG (Montagnard) and the RVN and some RF-PF (ethnic Vietnamese) forces. This was different. It was hard for us — for me — to assess for truth or relevance without reference to the American experience with our own minorities, with the indigenous red man, for example, and the black man. The accounts and claims ranged from the trivial to the serious.

The RVN soldiers look sloppy. The Montagnards smartly salute us. The RVN don't fight at night and are afraid to go on patrol around the airstrip.[3] This caused some problem recently. Apparently bombers hit near Hanoi and Haiphong and we expected a kind of retaliation. The Huey and observation planes which patrol at sun up and dusk thought they spotted a mortar position near the airstrip. The RVN troopers wouldn't go out for a look.

Montagnards have love and trust for Americans. They might kill a Vietnamese in a moment of rage but an American is safe with them. The Vietnamese in business will lie, cheat, and steal.

The Montagnards are better skilled laborers. A gentleman from California who is in Ban Me Thuot in his 3rd year as a civilian contractor tries to hire only Montagnards. They will work in a lumber yard and won't touch a scrap without asking permission. Permission is always granted.

Although they fight as mercenaries, I have it from the authority of advisors here that they make tough and loyal soldiers.

I had my own theory about such partisanship, such biased accounts. It was that either our collective guilt about our national policies towards our own indigenous peoples, or our identification with them as underdogs, was playing a role. Pvt. Rodriguez's experience is consistent with this. He writes:

I got attached to Rhade cause they were like me. I was raised in a very racist society against the so-called Mexican minority. Texans leave out the first three flags to describe us (Six Flags over Texas).[4] I had heard about the animosity between the Rhade and the Vietnamese, their belief that Vietnamese were their oppressors. I was raised that way [Alfonso Rodriguez, personal communication].

An interesting counterpoint appears in Charles Burns' self-published memoir, *Our War: Buon Ho, Vietnam 1966–67* (2008), wherein he describes the crowd that would show up for the showing of outdoor movies projected against the outside wall of the police station building. Montagnard troopers preferred American Westerns, always in English, and cheered the Indians. In the showing of episodes of the TV show *Combat*, they always cheered the Germans.

Northerners vs. Southerners: A Toxic Rivalry

There was, too, tension among ethnic Vietnamese, between those of the North and those of the South, that I became aware of during my tour. I initially imagined this as like the rivalry between Yale and Harvard colleges, a friendly rivalry, Hanoi representing more the ideological capital and Saigon, the commercial capital, for example. I was skeptical about whispers that it might be, in actuality, toxic. Mike Benge, in a recent communication, gives credence to the latter:

Probably the greatest factor [in diminishing the V.C. infrastructure] was the TET Offensive in which the NVA used the V.C. as cannon fodder to take the brunt of the causalities in order to take over the command of most V.C. units. The Northerners did not trust the Southerners and saw this as an opportunity to insert its Northern command structure into the V.C. units so they would have less to deal with when they took over the South. There was a continuous power struggle and purges within the Vietnamese Communist Party; e.g., the pro–Soviet communists got rid of many of the pro–Chinese at one stage of the game and then at another time, [it was] vice versa. The same with the Northerners against the Southerners [Mike Benge, personal communication].

I have not told anybody this. I knew a lot of Rhade that were associated with the FULRO. They were very anti–Communist and I was aware of their animosity towards the Vietnamese. Being Mexican, until I went in the Army I could sympathize with some of their arguments. I had just moved from Texas where there was much prejudice [Alfonso Rodriguez, personal communication].

6

Ban Me Thout:
An Unorthodox Practice

The hospital is very old, understaffed, poorly equipped, and over-crowded. Dr. Niem has been anxiously awaiting the MILPHAP Team for many months now. He delegates the care of patients — as is their custom — to technicians (3-year training course) and nurses (several months course).

The hospital is a series of yellowish stucco single floor buildings with patios interconnected by walks which have a roof supported by columns. The capacity is 200 beds but, as the patients occupy 2–3/bed, the census is considerably higher.

People use woven mats instead of mattresses. The wards are over-crowded, especially since relatives and family stay with the patients, feeding them, etc. Patients provide their own food. Families camp out under the beds, in the aisles, outside the building. Sanitation is a problem. One old lady and a sink is the "hospital laundry."

There are no latrines for the families living with the patients. Behind the surgery ward is a black, foul-smelling, fly-infested streamlet with pooled feces, urine and infected waste. It put other patients, not to mention visitors, families, and staff, at risk. As Pfc. Guingrich writes in a personal communication, "Parasitic infections were as common here as nails infestation in the tropics. Every single patient I performed a laboratory examination on had this disease and I, too, endured several bouts with parasitic infections for which we all regularly took a concoction of piperazine citrate during a 24-hour fast, the treatment for roundworm, Ascaris Lumbricoides."

The Frenchman who designed these structures evidently made no allowance for sharing or sanitation issues. Why not a large barbeque pit for families to use for cooking? A shelter for them to live in? A well for their water? People defecate outside the window. Why, since then, didn't anyone ever think to build a latrine or dig a pit or slit trench?

The pay wards are integrated, including both Montagnards and [ethnic] Vietnamese, an innovation. The charity wards are kept separate. The Montagnard charity patients are in an old garage with their children, chickens, cooking equipment. etc.

Maternity is entirely in the care of midwives. They consult a doctor only when they run into complications.

The entire hospital staff goes home from noon to 3:00 P.M. and everyone leaves at night. One technician for the hospital covers the other hours. Deliveries, surgery, emergencies, etc. must wait until the staff returns at 3:00 P.M. or the next morning. Until then people fend for themselves.

No one appears to take care of hospital grounds. The jungle grass and under-growth is slowly creeping up. You can almost see this place as it will look a year from now, abandoned.

Our equipment hasn't arrived yet. We're beginning to formulate a schedule, to be modified, of course, as the needs arise and as we become familiar with the people and the set-up.

After several tours and discussions we agreed on an initial deployment plan for our team. As I wrote, not all of the hospital buildings are ours. The greater section is military. They have better equipment, a surgeon, and a handsome budget. That's one of the big problems here; military has priority. 80 percent of Vietnam's doctors are in the army. That leaves one doctor for approximately 90,000 civilians and a skinny budget. They are further handicapped because renovations, etc. must be cleared through the province chief, usually a military man. Red tape prevents action. Even if he accedes, the minister of health in Saigon must approve. Frequently, letters aren't even answered.

I understand they plan to decentralize the Health Service. But the French bequeathed this system. It's hard to break a habit.

Our work is cut out for us. It'll be slow going, I'm sure, but we'll try not to be too ambitious and then disappointed. As a doctor I'll be working under handicaps I've never before imagined, language being but one of them. We certainly can't make the situation any worse than it is now.

I have a head cold now and had a touch of diarrhea yesterday. It's cool in the evenings and we sleep with blankets.

I intend, as soon as we are established in the hospital, wearing summer white shirt and going barefoot in sandals as Dr. Niem does.

Outpatient Clinic: First Patients

My assignment is outpatient clinic. I have a sergeant and private assigned to me and an interpreter. The day before beginning work we were

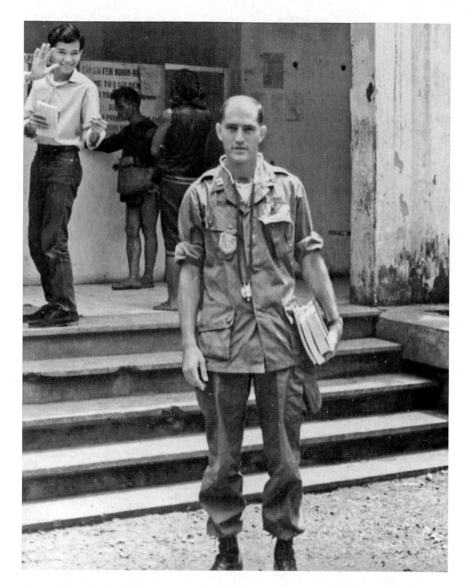

Outpatient clinic, Dar Lac province hospital (civilian side); Nguyen Hoan, interpreter (left rear), author (center), Montagnard patients register (in background).

standing on the hospital grounds and a Montagnard woman approached me. She had a goiter. She was dressed in the beautiful woven skirt, shawl covering her breasts, and a very unusual head piece — reminded me of pictures of women of Lapland. We found a Vietnamese to interpret. We explained that we wouldn't be set up to treat her for another week. But the Vietnamese doctor, a woman doctor from town who works mornings in the outpatient clinic, could see her here right away. She said she'd come back next week.

I attend clinic in jungle fatigues and boots. We walk to work because our jeeps haven't arrived.

The people line up with their animals, children, etc. and are registered on the porch. They come inside and a technician asks what is the matter. At most she will lean slightly forward in her seat to look at the wound, etc. and then prescribe. I can't imagine what she is writing. Then, the patient goes into the next room for a "shot." Everything is given by injection. Any patient the technician can't handle is sent to the civilian doctor or myself.

The technician and the Vietnamese civilian (woman) doctor were my advisees, my counterparts, in terms of my MACV mission. Interestingly, because the Vietnamese pronunciation of my name sounds similar to a directional anti-personnel fragmentation mine used by the U.S. military, "Claymore," they always giggled when speaking my name. I was happy to be just Bac Si ("Bok-see-ee").

My first patient was the wife of a leper driven in by Miss Aide who is senior technician (an American) at the leprosarium 14 kilometers outside of town. All their doctors had been kidnapped by the Vietcong 4 years ago and not heard from since. We don't go there because it's into the jungle and V.C. are hidden there. She spoke fluent Rhade but the patient spoke another dialect. The translation was accomplished and I wrote instructions for this woman who will return in a week. I'm curious to learn more of Miss Aide, the medical missionary. There are several young American women out there. Why did they come?

From my journal:

Why am I running? Because the Vietnamese youngster in my arms still breathes? Because I can't abide his dying in his father's arms waiting his turn to see me? Later I will hear of the murmurs. Who had ever seen a doctor running? Who had even heard of a doctor carrying his patient to the in-patient ward, let alone as the entire hospital was shutting down for the noon siesta? Nobody really expected the boy to live anyway. He had rabies. By mid–afternoon the boy is dead, the clinic up and operating again, and I am feeling disoriented.

From my journal:

I disqualify myself. The authorities simply have to find someone else to determine whether or not their prisoner is malingering. A Vietcong suspect, he apparently had a seizure during an interrogation. They need to know, because if he's not malingering they probably won't execute him.

Connections and Misfires II

Dr. Niem has had patients come in with notes from Vietcong medics asking us to take care of them as they haven't the facilities. (MILPHAP Teams from last fall have had similar referrals.)

If a Montagnard really likes you he will make you a blood-brother. The ceremony consists of getting drunk on their rice wine with the addition of blood of an ox that they have tethered in a field and slowly beaten to death. They feel that the more time it takes to die, the more time the spirit has to prepare for the next world. Then they present you with a brass bracelet.

Montagnards seem to have a different concept of time. You cannot get a chronology of a symptom. Either they've had the symptom "a long time" or "very long time." This, however, was through two interpreters. One translated Rhade to Vietnamese, the other from Vietnamese to English.

Everything is given by injection. The Vietnamese picked this up from the French. They don't take pills. A shot is good. A pill is nothing. Shots, shots, shots. This is one habit we expect to change.

A second habit picked up from the French is the prescription of camphor.[1] Our textbook in pharmacology lists no medical value for this.

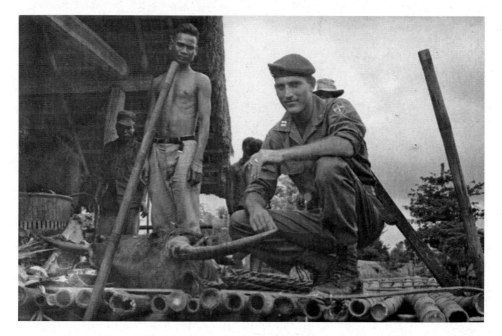

Author on deck of a Rhade longhouse. Note the head of a water buffalo, ceremonially sacrificed.

I admitted one young Montagnard boy with probably typhoid fever. There are several different diseases that may look like typhoid fever but the diagnosis is established by culturing the organism or by special test. We have no such lab facilities. If we can break down the possible diagnoses to half-dozen we're ready to start treatment. At best we can send a specimen to the Pasteur Institute in Saigon and get results in 4–5 weeks. The diagnosis would by then be academic. Anyhow, I wrote orders for chloramphenical (a broad-spectrum antibiotic).

I went to the hospital pharmacy and brought out a bottle and put it before the clerk who was writing out my orders in Vietnamese. Naturally, I asked that the boy be sent to the ward to which the American team had been assigned. After clinic I went to the ward to see the boy again. I checked the order the clerk had written. Camphor and Vitamin C by injection!

The needles are all dull, the IV tubing is used over and over, collecting dust on filthy shelves between times. Oh, God.

I throw away enough food everyday to feed my patients suffering malnutrition. Some have vitamin deficiencies, others have what our textbooks call, "famine," or "nutritional edema." So I saved food from the officers mess (hot dogs, vegetables, etc.) and brought it to a hospitalized Montagnard man with a huge belly and swollen hands and feet, and also to a young girl very low on red blood cells. It was to be their "medicine." But the hungry visitors, relatives and patients, gathered about me. One old lady held out her hands, begging. I really don't know if I caused more damage than good. I felt terrible.

The night technician must be given a separate set of instructions. They don't take orders from the patient's chart. After 4:00 P.M. orders must be written in a special book. If there is no drug in the hospital patients go into town and buy it. At the town drug store all medications are available like chewing gum. I could go on and on.

It is obvious that the most ubiquitous medical problem on the wards is malaria-related. It is also clear that patients come only when the illness is far advanced and then, at the early signs of improvement, treatment is discontinued. We sent for medical texts to help us.

Bill Baxley and I went to look in on a woman on the obstetrical service at the request of Captain Wheeler, the covering MACV doctor. At that OB service we made an incorrect diagnosis, but it wasn't of a patient. It was of the Vietnamese nurse on that service. When we initially appeared at the unit — led and managed by mid-wives; no doctors here — the Vietnamese nurse who was on duty in her Florence Nightingale–like outfit approached to be of assistance to us. We were able to learn the patient's vital signs and see her chart by using creative pantomime. (We knew no words in Vietnamese at this early stage.) When we were through and leaving there was a certain awkwardness about saying thank you and just being polite about leave-taking. I don't remember saying anything. Bill had better manners.

As we left the unit Bill nodded his head several times to the nurses and, holding up his right hand, said, "Waaall, thank ye." (Bill is from Georgia.) The Vietnamese nurse, not missing a beat, replied in accent-free English, "Think nothing of it."

My Problems with Number "35"

This morning a Chinese opium smoker attacked me like a dog in heat. Right there on the porch of the clinic. He started humping. I thought I'd break his neck. Nguyen Hoan, my interpreter, ran inside and grabbed his Vietnamese-English Medical phrase book and came out, rapidly racing through the pages. Then he pointed out the word, "insane." I knew. Like, I knew. I knew. Oh, boy, did I know.

The crazy Chinese opium smoker came back. Co Nam (Co is "Miss") came in and looked a little put-out. I went to where she gives injections with student nurses and found him with his trousers off and an erection and his hands holding a pack of obscene pictures. I shooed him out. Hoan tells me Co Nam is afraid.

The Chinese opium smoker came back again and had to be handcuffed by the police guard. He became abusive.

The Chinese opium smoker is no longer allowed in the clinic. Now he is standing outside my window and tossing in fruit, corn, and cinnamon apples. Like other lecherous men he is called "ba muoui lam" (phonetically "bah-mooey-lam") which is Vietnamese for number 35. It seems there is a Chinese game with 40 pieces, each piece representing an animal. Piece number 35, ba muoui lam, is Old Goat.

Invited to a Party

We, the officers of MILPHAP, were surprised and honored to be invited to a party the province chief was having for the deputy advisor to the RVN 23rd Division, Lt. Col. Ireland, who was about to leave for home. Because the invitation said "Suits" for dress code, Sergeant Strickland had to scope out and borrow someone's suit for me. The party was held at the town hall.

All the Vietnamese province administrators were there along with the senior advisory staff of the MACV 33rd Advisory Team. Mike Benge from USAID was there, too. I was glad when Dr. Niem, who was there, chose to sit with us MILPHAP officers.

Doctor Niem is lean and tall for a Vietnamese with good looking features and appearing younger than his 38 years. He is married with children. As different Vietnamese boys and girls appeared on stage to sing with drum and electric guitar backing, he translated. Most songs were about war. "Who will carve my name on his weapon now that my love has gone?" "Who will bring flowers from the jungle?" We spoke together about music and instruments, about history. He told me that An-nam and Annamese is the name the Chinese gave these people long ago. It means "pacified south," a term that has had a bad psychological effect. Viet-Nam means "people who have marched to the south." He taught me much.

We talked about the Japanese occupation. A new singer is on stage, the Rhade daughter of the deputy province chief in charge of Montagnard affairs. A bronze, beautiful, tall (5'4") girl in Western dress. She sang a popular American love song. I don't remember how it goes or it's title. I don't know how I looked but Dr. Niem looked at me and asked, "Are you homesick?" I told him, "Don't ask." Then, to my great surprise, the MC made an announcement (in Vietnamese, of course) but I caught the "Bac Si Niem." He was asking Dr. Niem to come up and sing before these 60 dignitaries! As he rose to go up front he commented to me, "I don't remember any songs."

Doctor Niem apologized that he knew only one song, a sad song, and sang the most beautiful lament. No question, he was the best singer. When he returned to our table I shook his hand and asked if he played any instrument. He said, yes, the guitar. Not electric but "Spanish." In answer to his question I told him that I, too, played the guitar.

At the end of that evening he asked how I spent my evening hours. I told him reading and writing. "With all the leisure time you will have," he remarked, "that probably won't be enough. I know the people are slow to action and temporize." I hope one day to visit his home and get to know him better and more personally.

A messenger interrupted the party to let us know that 20 kilometers to the northwest an outpost alongside a refugee camp was under mortar attack. The advisors and province people left immediately.

Dr. Niem also shared a Vietnamese legend about the origins of the Montagnard race. According to that legend, many thousands of years ago a prince married a girl and she laid 100 eggs. Of the offspring, 50 went to the mountains, 50 to the coast.

Tradition or Personality:
Dancing with "Trickster"

We were there to augment — at least, assist with — the healthcare provided to Vietnamese civilians. We were not there to reform practices or make people do things differently. This was supposed to be win-win, good guys helping good guys. But we didn't hit the ground running. We didn't even hit the ground walking. We hit the ground stumbling and bumping into one another. Some of the people we were "assisting" seemed to us either professionally incompetent (by our standards) or with dysfunctional personality issues. Which was it, training or personality, the system or the person? Should we conform to their standards and, in so doing, fail to provide optimal care? Or reform that system at the cost of a collegial relationship? Something was broken and in need of fixing, in need of healing. It seemed that simple, only it wasn't. This was our conundrum. (Because the French had never prepared the Vietnamese people for any administrative leadership positions — they had never prepared the people for true independence — healthcare workers that graduated after 1956 when the French left must have received what I'd call substandard training. It was as if there was as yet no tradition of responsibility modeled by administrator-teachers.) For me, it was like dancing with that iconic figure of mythology, the Trickster. Every time we adhered to our military objective we'd be suborning our oath as physicians. Every time we adhered to our oath as physicians we'd be suborning our military mission. In either case, either our counterpart or a patient would also take the hit. Lose-lose.

Stan came to me in outpatient clinic. "Larry, got a minute? I've got to talk to you." We walked back to the office assigned the MILPHAP Team and he sat behind the desk. I relaxed in a chair and Lt. Brown slumped into the other chair. Stan began talking in a very slow, terse, deliberate way, trying hard to keep control. It seems he asked the nurse to draw blood for hemogram studies. She smiled and said, yes. Later in the afternoon, it was still not done. "Now," he said. To the interpreter he added, "Tell her I want it done NOW." The next day, after Dr. Niem had heard both sides, he told us her explanation for her behavior. "But I didn't think it was necessary to be done right away." Dr. Niem explained to this nurse that when the doctor gives an order the nurse doesn't question it. OK, that was one part of it. Then Stan changed the order to chloramphenical and said to give it. She smiled and wouldn't move. Later on she said she gave it. The mother of the patient said she hadn't. Then, she said they didn't have it in the hospital. Stan went back and produced a hand full of vials. He thrust them before her. Next morning, need I say, she got, not chloramphenical, but penicillin!

After Stan blew off steam we discussed how to handle it. Stan was for telling Dr. Niem. I objected because, in his speech before the staff Dr. Niem had emphasized the importance of interpersonal differences being settled between the parties involved "in the spirit of friendship and cooperation." We made up our minds to load the ward with MILPHAP'ers and carry out our own orders. Lt. Brown brought up the important point of rapport. Our instructions at Fort Sam were that we NOT take over a ward, etc. We had to teach the people to improve so as not to leave a vacuum when we left.

Sgt. Strickland, assigned to Stan's ward, has made a point of simply getting friendly with the nurses there. So work will get done and the Vietnamese staff will continue to be included.

As a touching sequel to the story of Stan and his head-strong nurse, as we left the office together a crowd of children ran after us shouting the only English they apparently knew, but, under the circumstances, it was a bad joke. They shouted, "O.K.! Number 10! O.K.! Number 10!" (We know, kid. Don't rub it in.)

I sat on my ass most of this morning. The civilian doctor showed up for 5 minutes. Most of the time there weren't any patients. I asked the technician, my counter-part, whether it was a busy morning. "Yes. Very, very busy." Is she kidding? They go home from noon to 3:00 p.m., work from 3:00 to 5:00. They move at a very slow pace. We had been drilled not to be ambitious. To suggest changes, then drop the subject. Mention it again several months later. Don't be impatient. Meanwhile, we might construct sanitary facilities outside the wards. If the relatives can be taught sanitation, especially outside the ward, we'll have an easier time introducing sanitation inside the ward itself. When I mentioned this suggestion, what I had in mind was, like, right now. Dr. Niem said, "Yes. It is a problem. After a while when you are settled in and we work together for a while we'll discuss this again." So, here is American know-how and muscle power smack against the tempo of tropical areas plus the importance of saving face. How can I suggest a change without implying that the existing conditions aren't good?

We are up against customs like lousy sanitation habits, traditions where a family comes and camps out in the hospital, poor methods where nurses are used to running a ward, to say nothing of the language barrier, no equipment, no drugs, a laboratory that sends patients home to produce their stool for examination while, outside their window, people produce samples on the grass. And the lab does tests tomorrow that can be done now in 30 minutes. There is a budget not worth shit. There is administrative red-tape which keeps the best qualified and most intelligent making out report after report. Frustration? I never heard of it before coming here.

Work with your counterparts, we were told. Do not attempt to take charge or to make changes. Avoid giving the impression that you know better. The ultimate goal of the MILPHAP mission seemed so clear back at Fort Sam. We were there to win the hearts and minds of the people to their government, not to ours. But making it clear did not make it doable.

We've begun a wash-down program. After stealing, etc. mops, Borax, and other cleaning items we've begun to swab down that ward. Our goal is to wash and air the mats, clean beds, wash patients' filthy clothes, and so on. But the patients continue to defecate on the porch. The kids — my typhoid case ... his urine is infectious ... began to urinate. The stream lifted gently in an arc and pooled on the mat, seeping into the weaving. His mother quickly gathered his shirt, her shawl and other wearing apparel to catch the urine.

The men working with Stan Banach took some mops and pails and went to work on the small 2-bed room next to the ward. Good job. When they left the patients on the ward asked us to leave the equipment behind. Next morning the pay ward was spanking clean.

In a small, unused closet-sized room in the outpatient clinic, we set up a treatment room. Here we are able to wash and apply ointment to diseased skin, sponge patients burning with fever, give enemas for constipation and set up intravenous fluids. We give ear irrigations, foot soaks and tapeworm purges. We apply skin creams.

Stan's days are one crisis after another. His interpreter is a nervous and not too fluent young man who says, "Yes, yes" and that's all. Stan asked him to ask a patient when he had urinated last. The reply: "He say his father die last year."

Stan ordered 0.25 grains or 15 mg of phenobarbital to be given twice daily to a convulsing febrile child. The next morning the child's mother said her baby wouldn't wake up. Stan asked the nurse to show him how much phenobarbital she'd given the child. It amounted to almost 200 mg twice daily when his order was maximum 15 mg twice daily. The baby never woke up. She died.

Nurses don't follow Stan's orders, add their own medications arbitrarily, and don't do anything "now." I was looking over a jaundiced man I had just admitted when Stan called me over. Another patient had aspirated (breathed in some gunk he'd coughed up; the danger is suffocation or pneumonia) and Stan wanted to perform a trach (open the windpipe). I jerked out my boy scout knife from my belt and grabbed some alcohol sponges. But the patient was bringing the stuff back up. So I cut a piece of the tubing from an IV setup and we passed it into his trachea to suck him out. The nurses stood around. They didn't do anything. We asked for this and that. Nothing.

I sit in outpatient clinic with my men and Hoan. The technician, my counterpart, sends patients into the hospital and Stan gets them without history, physical exam, or diagnosis but, of course, with an order for camphor and vitamin C. I wait and wait for my technician or doctor counterpart to send a patient to me. Once or twice during the morning she'll ask me to look at a particularly sick patient. Once she does I strip the (male) patient to his shorts and my men bring him outside for a wash down and then I examine him by the window where the light is good. Today I got bold. I asked to move the examining table to where there was optimal light, with their permission of course. My doctor-counterpart agreed. When we moved the examining table lots of little flies and worms emerged. Before you could say, "Civic Action," the table was in pieces outside and my men were making for the mops and Borax. Before they came back the Mountagnard clerk was washing the table and the people in pharmacy and the injection room were hurrying about sweeping and mopping their own rooms. Was it the stimulus of our action? Was it the sudden presence of mops and buckets? Was it "saving face"?

We had the room spic and span and I rearranged all the furniture so the examination area wasn't screened off and in the dark corner. It was placed before the huge screen-less window with lots of natural light. I set the "desks" (old, rotten tables) in rows giving a streamline appearance. I took, myself, to hand washing the filthy, dirty curtain we'd been using to screen off the examining area for privacy. Hoan, my interpreter, a handsome and soft spoken 20 year-old who'd given up his dream of becoming a pilot and elected law school instead but, that being untenable as well, took the position offered by USAID as interpreter, busily helped us moving furniture, etc. As I was working I commented, "You were hired as an interpreter. You don't have to do this." "You are a doctor and you are scrubbing linen," he pointed out. He is comfortable telling me when he doesn't understand something. He is constantly looking up new words in his dictionary. He plays guitar and we reviewed songs-in-common. They are, Red River Valley, Jingle Bells, Streets of Laredo, and many French songs. He's intelligent. He understands toxin and antitoxin, how they work. When he drew a cross-section of the spinal cord and labeled neuron tracks I was speechless.

Hoan doesn't translate my questions and comments. Instead I discuss with him the problem, anything from a patient's history to how to get into the pharmacy for inventory without shaming anyone. He grasps the problem and "interprets" for me and, thus, avoids the culture gap. While I walked through a Montagnard ward questioning patients about their problems I

*picked up some of their Vietnamese phrases and words, like for "headache"
and "for how long." Hoan remarked, "You have a good ear." I sense a friendship growing. And when the clinic is empty I try, try, try to break the ice
with my counterparts, the technician and the doctor. Hoan is very helpful
here. So far my counterparts have neither greeted me nor spoken to me first.*

*In the way of gentle pressure I told the technician that, as I have no
experience in tropical diseases, I'd appreciate her calling me over for interesting symptoms or lesions so I can learn from her. Of course, you know
damn well I don't trust what she does and want desperately to know what
the hell she is giving these poor people, let alone what she thinks is wrong
with them. She did let me look at a boy who probably has plague. I took
his note (patients keep their own paperwork) and wrote in English a brief
history, physical, lab tests, and medicine. I wanted him admitted. So she,
by my stimulus or to save face, for the first time actually bothered to write
something about the patient before sending him back to a ward. What she
wrote (in French) was adenopathie [adenopathy or swollen glands] of max-
illary region. Well, the maxilla is the cheek bone and the kids lump was
along his neck, his cervical region. I told her this. Then, with a straight
face, she told me I was wrong. I dropped the subject.*

*We picked up needles, gauze, zephiran [benzalkonium chloride, a top-
ical antiseptic] from the 155th Aviation Company and I passed them out in
outpatient clinic to the technicians. The place looks changed. This, because
of the spring cleaning and new arrangement of desks and chairs.*

*I'm still riding on the wave of optimism and excitement that has carried
me this far. But the slump will come when I look around and see what has
been accomplished.*

*Time flies by quickly. I get bored reading medicine. Chess gives me
comfort and distraction.*

When Ethical Imperatives Collide: My Tipping Point

I reached my tipping point. I let my prime directive as a physician (that
I do no harm) override my prime directive as a military officer (that I not
take over and attempt to reform this dysfunctional healthcare system). The
issue was the customary outpatient practice of bypassing an actual examination
or input by a doctor. There was nothing special about this particular case. It
was more that my passive acquiescence suddenly felt egregious. It was as if,
as a docile bystander, I was enabling something harmful. (It followed on the
heels of a patient dying.)

Several days ago my technician counterpart admitted a wrinkled and cold, sick old lady. The technician never asked me to examine the patient although I was sitting and doing nothing six feet away from her. Her diagnosis was cholera. I visited the patient that afternoon and mulled over the case all weekend. Come Sunday I was seriously considering the alternative diagnosis of algid malaria. It, too, dries people up and makes them cold. With cholera you give saline solution intravenously. When you do they live. When you don't they die. I knew all weekend she was getting Ringer's lactate solution because they were out of the saline solution and they figure that any solution is better than none. On the way to work today I debated over and over how best to indicate to the technician that patients sick enough to be admitted warrant a doctor's consultation. She mustn't lose face; I understand that. But this had gone far enough.

The solution came easier than I anticipated. The old lady died over the weekend. I sat with my teammates watching this counterpart glibly treating people without making a diagnosis. Then, suddenly, a baby was being carried out the back door towards the wards. She was doing it again! She was admitting a patient without my even being asked to take a look. I raced after the father and led him and the baby he was carrying back to the clinic. I was mad and didn't give a damn about people losing face. I tore up her admission slip with her medications and wrote one of my own.

What followed was the most productive morning and afternoon. I was flooded with patients. My men set to work. I saw malaria, hookworm, dengue fever, plague, impetigo, diphtheria, goiter, and countless unknowns. My men were scrubbing everybody and their relatives and children and cleaning skin sores. Word was spreading and patients hospitalized for days and weeks dragged themselves off the wards to come to the outpatient clinic for me to see them.

The technician was quite subdued. She was not unfriendly, considering. In the afternoon, between 2 o'clock and 5 o'clock there are generally no patients although the clinic is officially open. There was a mob when I returned from lunch. When the civilian doctor [my other counterpart] arrived she took one look and turned around and left. I called out to her to return. She said something about seeing the wards.

While my counterpart may have been bent out of shape, it seemed our healthcare setting had suddenly become more vital. The hospital was even recovering some of its earlier reputation. Morale was picking up and patients were feeling better. The tradeoff? The hearts and minds of the people had just been pushed the wrong way. What I was doing was exactly what I'd been enjoined from doing by my military superiors. I was not seeing the forest for the trees because the trees were people. But I felt good about it.

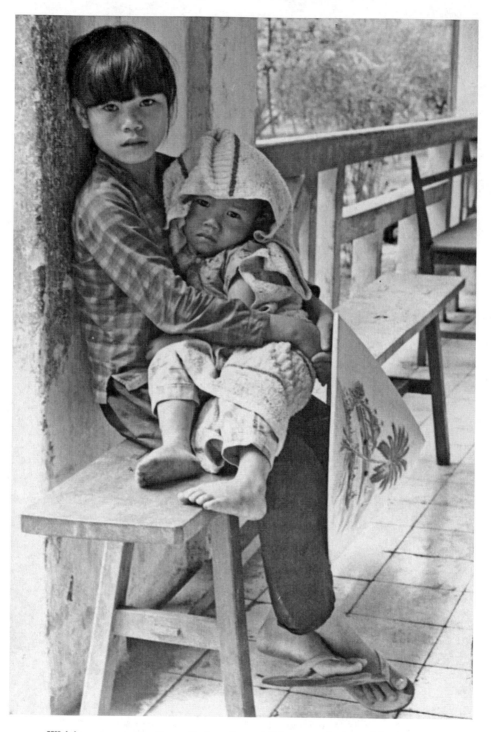

Waiting area, outpatient clinic, where children touch you with their eyes.

"Welcome to the Club"

The police came to the hospital Friday to tell us that their agents in town have heard that the Vietcong plan to grenade the MILPHAP Team. We told him, thank you. I was among the last to leave for home. I walked with Sergeant Sanders who works in the clinic with me. We walked on opposite sides of the road. All the time I'm listening to the bikes coming up behind me and the motor scooters, checking my rear without seeming obvious. I was also selecting the ditches that would be good for jumping into and trees good for running behind. On the home stretch the road was crowded with bulls and cows and just past them a body lay prone in the street.

As Sanders and I approached we took turns shouting, "Hey, get up!," "Hey, you. Get up!" Nothing. We didn't stop. As we drew near we saw it was a shepherd boy sleeping. Not unusual, apparently.

Back at the Bungalow we told Mike Benge and the advisers. Their only comment was, "Welcome to the Club." Apparently, this is standard operating procedure for the V.C. Nothing ever comes of it.

Later we practiced firing our weapons out at the RF-PF Training Camp outside of town.

Unable to See the Forest for the Trees
Because the Trees Are People

I'm upset and frustrated and needing to talk it out. This morning in outpatient clinic I sat four and a half hours seeing 25 patients, my record to date considering having everything translated. The technician turned all the patients over to me and left. The civilian doctor came and saw 2 or 3 patients and then she, too, left. As lunch hour approached the nurses and staff on the wards left and locked up their offices along with the medicine and equipment. The pharmacist left and locked up. The administrator who fills out admission forms left. Meanwhile my men and myself were admitting a year-old baby with tetanus. His jaw is locked and he whines as he tries to grip mama's nipple in his mouth. Also, a man burning with typhoid fever, a pale woman who we carried to the ward by stretcher — her blood count must be near zero — a man with jaundice and fever, possibly black-water fever, a fatal complication of malaria.

I planned to by-pass doing laboratory tests as they, too, were locked up for the weekend and, after lunch, take one man and my interpreter and shake the keys from the permanent technician and go to the ward and give intravenous, give anti-sera, sponge down the babies myself. The permanent technician says he has no keys and all medications are locked up. I asked for erythromycin for the girl with amoebiasis. He says there is no erythromycin. But I'd seen it on the shelf in the pharmacy just yesterday! Same for penicillin, tetracyclines, etc. It's there on the shelves but they deny this.

The pharmacy, by the way, is run by Vietnamese personnel who are reluctant to let us look around. They don't cooperate and won't relinquish their authority. I've prescribed a drug, griseofulvin, for children with ringworm. But, rather than send the kid back with a note saying they don't have griseofulvin, they prescribe, at the same dosage, a sulfa drug or other arbitrary antibiotic which could possibly cause severe damage.

As I sit here typing I know my little lockjaw baby will probably die and the man with typhoid fever develop complications such as a perforated intestine, common in Vietnam, and the anemic lady will go downhill and the man with blackwater fever will also die. But the medicine is here. Only the system won't let us have it. And, the sad part is that, when these people die, their relatives don't feel bitter or angry. They don't know that the patient had a chance. It makes me sick.

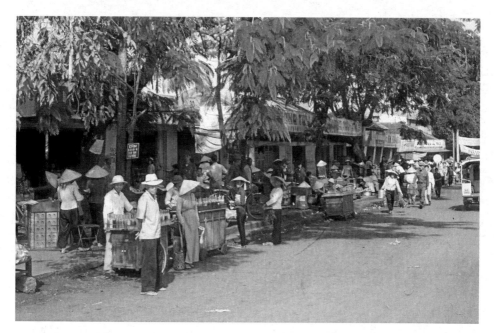

The commercial pharmacy was located in the center of Ban Me Thuot where soldiers, civilians, ethnic Vietnamese, Montagnards and Americans mingled and shopped for items both legitimate and black market. (Doctor-prescriptions were not necessary at the pharmacy.)

I ask relatives of a patient to buy a liter of dextrose and water in town for an intravenous. They pay twice the rate, get half a liter and add two vials of medicine a friend once used for another illness. They have injected two vials before I discover this. It is sodothiol and isn't in any of our books.

If the pharmacy didn't have a specific medicine, the technician selected another they did have and dispensed it in the dose indicated for the original.

Available statistics estimated that 50 percent of the children born didn't live to age five. Average life expectancy was less than 40.

USAID provided powdered milk, wheat and protein supplements for exclusive use on the Montagnard charity ward.

There was a report of an epidemic at a Dar Lac village with 40 deaths. There were no choppers available over the weekend. Stan and Capt. Wheeler went out there today. False alarm.

A follow-up on my baby with lockjaw. I went to see him today but his mother had taken him away. Without my interpreter I had no way of knowing if he was dead or had received the anti-toxin and pulled through.

Culture Clash: The Rhade Story

This was Montagnard ancestral land. What was their story, here in Dar Lac? Benge, in his article about the Montagnards,[2] introduces them. The Montagnards, he explains, were a people who had evolved in relationship with their surroundings and had lived, in their view, in harmony with the spirits of the elements. They farmed the slopes and bottomland within the cycle of the rainy season, clearing, planting, and fallowing their fields until yields decreased; then new fields were cleared and the cycle resumed. They drew water, fished, bathed, and washed clothes in nearby streams. Forests provided game, wild fruits and vegetables, dyes to color their cotton cloth, medicines and firewood. The forests also provided grasses, hardwood, bamboo, and rattan for houses and artifacts.

Here, in Dar Lac, the Montagnard people lived in raised longhouses as extended families "where the younger generation learned by observation and oral presentation the culture, customs, mores, values, and history of their people. Occasionally, one could find a few smaller individual or dual-family houses interspersed among the longhouses in villages. In societies with matrilineal decent, the longhouse, land, and other properties are owned by the women."

French colonial policy had kept the Montagnards and ethnic Vietnamese apart but, in 1954, Diem's regime attempted to assimilate the Montagnards by abolishing tribal schools and courts and introducing 200,000 ethnic Vietnamese into the hills, often violating tribal tenure rights. The appointed Vietnamese province chief decreed the Montagnards must wear shirts and slacks. In Pleiku they were forbidden to build their homes off the ground. Women were enjoined from going bare-breasted. All of this contributed to their nationalist underground movement, FULRO.

In the early 1960s, one attempt by Americans and Vietnamese to win the allegiance of the tribes, the Village Defense Program, in Dar Lac (see, Chapter 1) had immediate and striking success. A Special Forces team of twelve army men and two civilians, with backing from the CIA, had, at that time, begun to instruct Rhade men, at their camp several miles to the northeast of Ban Me Thuot, on how to fire modern weapons, watch trails, and conduct counter-ambushes. More Rhade men showed up and wanted to learn. By the end of 1962 there were multiple newly constructed Rhade villages featuring a protective force of 400 Rhade soldiers, always on patrol outside the villages. These forces were mercenaries and were designated Civilian Irregular Defense Group (CIDG) forces, called "strikers" by the U.S. Special Forces who'd trained and led them. Ethnic Vietnamese Special Forces, the counterparts of these U.S. Special Forces advisors, were, in time, to assume their leadership when the Americans moved on. By the end of 1972 this CIDG program had 200 Montagnard villages with a population of around 60,000 protected by 1,500 trained Montagnard Strike Force soldiers. (Approximately 50 of the 80-plus A-team camps in Vietnam had Montagnard troops.)

Unfortunately, when the Americans stepped back and moved on and let the Vietnamese Special Forces officers take full command, the traditional antipathy of Vietnamese to the tribes and tribal distrust of the Vietnamese resurfaced.[3] Those Special Forces camps, absent Americans, fell apart. The Rhade left and the numbers of tribesmen on the government side began falling. This was the situation that led up to the Montagnard revolt in 1964, two years before I arrived. I was able to discover no specific tipping point. Mike Benge, who was there, remembers it this way:

> While the Americans were in command of a Special Forces camp, there was a shadow command of Vietnamese Special Forces troops, who often refused to go along with patrols and fight the V.C., were arrogant toward the Montagnard CIDG forces, and often crooked and tied-in with corrupt Vietnamese contractors who furnished supplies and food to the camps. Also, there were cases of corruption among the Vietnamese pay masters who cheated the Montagnards and their families) including payment of indemnification funds for wounded, crippled and killed CIDG forces [personal communication].

When I showed up in Ban Me Thuot in 1966, I knew nothing of this history or of the rebellion, let alone its causes and impact, even as its impact and meaning was assuredly in the memory of everyone there, ethnic Vietnamese and Montagnard alike. It was certainly in the memory of the Rhade. Then I began working with Rhade as healthcare colleagues and as patients coming to the clinic for medical attention and, later, as Special Forces strikers who, from time to time, would provide security when I traveled into villages and hamlets.

Would it have made a difference had I'd known this story and how intercultural relations between the ethnic Vietnamese and Montagnard had cut so deeply? Would I have recognized my own stumbling experience and unwitting offenses in that story? But I was a healer. My medicine was "good" medicine. Then, again, I'd read *The Ugly American*, the 1958 novel by Burdick and Lederer, and knew that the villain of that fictional story looked like me.

Corruption, Elephant in the Room

One subtext to the Vietnamese healthcare system's mission, another agenda that was below our radar, was slow coming into focus for me. Yes, change takes time, and this is largely because the people who will be doing the changing need time to come around and own it; change works best when the person owns it. And sometimes, when one is depleted, one just can't think of "owning" yet one more thing. But I don't believe that was the only subtext going on. It was, as if, on some level, there was an additional issue about ensuring the stability of the existing system and the people in it, an issue that would impact the effectiveness of our mission, namely, maintaining the status quo, the broken status quo. The corrupted status quo. Given the frequent leadership changes and uncertainty about just about everything, I should have been able to appreciate everyone's need in Vietnam simply to "stay on course," which meant resisting all the pushes and pulls, the jerks and bounces that thrust you this way and that way, and just "holding on." And what one held on to, for better or for worse, would be one's resources and one's ways, what one had and what was familiar. The Vietnamese military system had a reputation for this. You conserved what you had; you didn't spend it, waste it, or drop it. So why should the public health system be different? Corruption takes different forms.

But I never considered this. I never considered the many politicians and military people and *their* systems and agendas. I never gave thought to the politicking necessary to maintaining any position with two heads, one military and one civilian. I was barely aware that Doctor Niem's might be a balancing act obliging mindfulness of multiple agendas. Here's one example: What could be more important to a hospital administration than improved or optimal care? Here's what: needing to hold on to staff, to keep the peace and stay in business and, now, to keep MILPHAP from leaving. Besides, what was the actual reach of Doctor Niem's role and mandate anyway, considering there was no possibility for oversight or dismissal? He knew his MILPHAP Team were under orders not to take over, and he was desperate that we gain a foothold as well as that he keep his staff. He understood the big picture and his was the long-view. He saw the forest. I liked, respected, and trusted Dr. Niem but, unlike him, I was impatient. The people and their personal distress were in *my* face, everyday, not his, and I couldn't see beyond the trees. We Americans counted days as if our lives depended on it whereas the Vietnamese, I found, were not that short-sighted. (And their lives did depend on it.)

I was, back in 1966, very much at the start of a very steep learning curve and had barely moved up a bit when it came time for me to leave. But the traction I found there did prove durable and my memories from that time encouraged progress up that curve the rest of my life. Ironically, I found the same issues, the same competing priorities and covert agendas back home, and the same risk of doctor burn-out, but with a difference: back home, the risk of burnout was not lethal.

Warily Co-Existing with Murmurs of Success

Waiting for our equipment to arrive was, potentially, a time of relationship-building, at least a time of wary co-existing. Sometimes we made friends, sometimes not.

I love to watch the children looking after one another, the older ones playing mother to the younger ones as is their custom. As a matter of fact, when a girl comes with a baby on her hip I never know if she's "mama" or "big sister." Hoan knows but I still can't pick correct ages.

Mornings are livened up sometimes by that crazy Chinese man who, no longer allowed in the clinic, still comes outside my window and tosses in fruit, cinnamon apples, corn, and other "gifts" which Hoan tosses back out.

I have the unique opportunity to observe typhoid fever run its natural course without being altered by medicine. The young girl has burning fever and a terrific headache plus the characteristic red spots. She'll suffer this severe toxemia for longer than a week before it slowly remits. I don't remember the odds for her survival. The drug, chloramphenical, is specific and will cure her. But doctors and technicians give everybody with fever all kinds of antibiotics so when the specific need arises, they're out of the one you need. The supply situation was critical when we arrived. Scrounging from other people we've beefed up the drug supply to keep the hospital going. They were about to be all washed up as a hospital at the time of our arrival. Now, our meager contributions are almost gone. If we don't have supplies within a week, it'll be over. Without antibiotics the place is lost.

About that gal with typhoid fever, I discovered some samples of aspirin mailed to me at Fort Sam so I gave her two. (No medicines are dispensed on weekends.) Stan's patient with malaria continues to spike daily temps to 105 degrees. We were about to switch her from chloroquine to quinine when he discovered the nurse hadn't been giving him his chloroquine. Two seriously ill patients left this weekend without being given medications that we do have. We make rounds on weekends but, as the pharmacy as well as offices are locked, we can only watch as patients go downhill.

A good week. I treated more patients than previous weeks. Stan had no deaths on his ward. (But his string of five days without a patient walking out was broken this weekend when those two I'd mentioned walked out for lack of treatment.) We still don't have a functioning lab.

We doctors and Lt. Brown met with Dr. Niem, along with the civilian lady doctor who works in the clinic with me, and the military surgeon, who has helped at the civilian hospital. We told Dr. Niem of the lack of cooperation from hospital staff and the lack of treatment at night on weekends, etc. When Stan's nurse was called in for an accounting and lied Stan told her to her face she was lying. Dr. Niem promised action.

Lt. Col. Monroe, who replaced Lt. Col. Ireland as 2nd in command for the 33rd Advisory Team, toured the hospital. He nearly hit the ceiling. He couldn't believe his eyes. He's hot to organize a tour or inspection with some big wheels in Saigon.

Saturday we met with Dr. Jackson, a civilian, the Director of Medicine for II Corps Area, and a representative of Gen. Humphreys who oversees MILPHAP. Lt. Col. Monroe was there. They gasped at some of our stories. They'll stay several days to write a separate report. They kept telling us things were better since we arrived, that people were being cured and word was spreading, that people were bringing their friends and families in for treatment. They also promised action. We won't last more than a week with the medications at hand.

Lt. Col. Monroe is concerned about the hospital but even more so about the outlying districts. He realizes that soldiers aren't enough to win the people over. We've been trained in counter-insurgency. If he can supply security I am now more than eager to hit the road. I know we can work wonders with the Montagnards in their villages. They respond.

The Patient Was Vietcong

Hoan, sits with me in clinic and spots Vietcong for me. Some are clandestine. He recognizes their outfits and sandals. (Hoan is, himself, from the North.) Other times they are North Vietnamese deserters who have accepted the South's "Open Arms" Policy wherein they turn themselves in, go for rehabilitation, and then are let go. They are undernourished, tired, worried about their sick kids, just like any of the fathers coming to the clinic with their children.

I saw our first case of confirmed vivax malaria. Falciparum is the Central Highland species. Vivax is in the Mekong Delta and along the coast. This patient denies leaving Ban Me Thuot. Treatment is the same so no problem but it will make interesting reading for readers of our MILPHAP Report.

I am embarrassed now to admit that, at such moments back then, I used to have brief conversations with myself and wonder if other soldiers didn't have similar internal conversations. The conversation would be done in a flash but it had a lasting effect. Slowed down, these conversations went like this. (To myself) "My God. This is an enemy soldier. I'm looking at him and talking to him. I'm going to help him now. But he doesn't look evil. Is this one a Vietcong terrorist?" Then I'd think, "I'm a tough American. Surely I'm worthy of an enemy more substantial than this sick, tired, worried, small fellow." Something didn't compute and I couldn't make it compute. So I concluded, "His commanding officer must be the evil one, the terrorist. Yes. That's it." But I was always left with the unmilitary, if not unmanly and puzzling, epiphany that I couldn't imagine myself killing him because I couldn't picture him killing anyone. Was I wrong to conclude that he wasn't a monster? And that neither was I?

I Am the Ugly American

Reading my letters I wonder: how was I not a bully and insensitive, arrogant and insulting? I was sounding like one, to read my letters home. I was hurtful, me, an officer and a doctor.

How to improve the outpatient clinic? The technician must go. The Vietnamese technician prescribes camphor and Vitamin C to everyone; no history, physical exam, or diagnosis. She admits patients without consulting with me. I repeatedly ask her to consult with me. She asks me to bring her paper cups and gauze compresses for her to take home but I've told her that these items we've brought in we'd bought with our own money.

This filthy mess of buildings shaded by great tropical trees and uncut grass with chickens and dogs running everywhere and half-naked people squatting by outdoor fires and children who don't even interrupt their play to urinate and foul their naked legs—this "hospital" is rotten. And we're obliged to augment existing facilities which means working with people, some of whom have the attitude of tyrannical petty officials.

An hysterical woman with multiple human teeth bites on her body came in with her policeman son. She wanted to be admitted. The technician wrote for chest X-Ray and antibiotics and more. I called her back, examined her, and, over the objections of her son, refused admission. She received tetanus anti-toxin which was all she needed.

Everyone's on a Learning Curve

People are coming in increasing numbers. Add to my list of diseases treated: tapeworm, trichimoniasis, rabbit-plague (in humans), drownings (now that monsoon rains have been increasing), maggots, and fevers of unknown origin (FUOs). Also plague (but after two days on streptomycin they look like a million dollars), malaria with its' characteristic periodicity with fever and chills, jaundice from infectious hepatitis, malaria, Weil's Disease [also known as Liptospirosis, transmitted to people from animals, primarily rats and mice].

Tetanus is common. The ones with pneumonia go right under. Heart disease is almost unknown.

There was a hell of a storm several nights back. The monsoons are coming down and we're beginning to see the consequences. The morning after the big rain when 5 inches fell, a family of 7 was brought to the hospital. All wet, blue, and quite drowned; the entire family wiped out. I couldn't understand how people drown in a rainstorm even though a child drowned just last week. So I drove with Hoan to the neighborhood where it happened. Then I knew. A very deep ravine, at least 7 feet deep with slimy mud walls cut into a very steep hillside. Shacks were crowded on either side and also over the ravine supported by stilts. Rooms opened up onto this ravine. People could stand in the living rooms and toss garbage into the pit, toss waste. During heavy rains this gully fills up with fast moving rapids. If a pillar is knocked out an entire room falls below to be swept 500 feet down the hillside. I don't know what really happened to that family of 7 but that place is a trap.

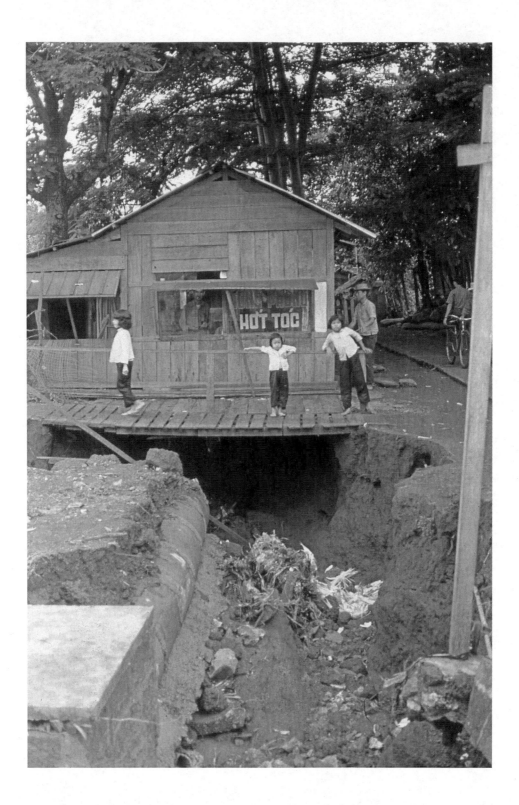

Right now, sitting in the hospital office typing, two small girls with their brothers on their hips, have come to keep me company. I drew them some cartoons. We're friends.

Our jeeps and equipment have arrived. Someone scratched the parasitology books and tropical medicine texts off the list. Now we've got $1,500 worth of books on oral surgery, anatomy, administrative texts, and group psychiatry. But I got one on skin diseases and one on pediatrics. The USAID people give us powdered milk and wheat and protein supplements for exclusive use on the Montagnard charity ward. The colonel in command of the 33rd Advisory Team is working on projects to renovate here, to build shelters and cookouts for families of patients and build sanitary facilities.

Cases of vivax malaria begin appearing. Not uncommonly this follows heavy fighting in the Mekong Delta 200 miles to the southwest. Sector is interested. Malaria in the Central Highlands is always the falciparum type.

It is very common to see fever, headache, and cough with abdominal pain. This could be anything. Four patients had these complaints and developed pink, raised, discrete and blanch-able spots between the umbilicus and nipples. We all agreed, typhoid fever, and gave aspirin. We're out of chloramphenicol. Now they have this rash on their extremities and face but not the back. What is it? Dengue? But that rash is confluent. Typhus? But that disease causes petechiae and axillary involvement. We're in the dark.

We've been visited by a World Health Organization (WHO) man, an old French doctor, who has been here most of his life. He makes inspection tours of lab facilities. His was a quick stop. He looked in on our lab and said, "Zero."

In outpatient clinic there is an adjoining room with tile counter, sink, cabinet, and bed that had been dusty and unused. We set it up as a treatment room, the idea being to expand outpatient facilities and encourage the Vietnamese workers to give more care than Vitamin C injections. I was informed yesterday that the night technician doesn't want us to use "his" room. We'll move out. There is another large, unused room with running water. We'll build an examining table there and buy a screen of mats. If my technician counterpart ever avails herself of my men and our treatments I'll make my first notch in my desk to honor such a visible advance.

My spirits have taken a lift since our equipment began coming in. My clinic is doing booming business. I'm rested, well-fed, and looking forward to some improvements.

Opposite: It was into this deep crevasse that passed beneath so many houses as it cut down the hillside that a family drowned during August monsoon rains.

I'd like to lay my hands on the drugs used by the Chinese Medicine Man. I no longer consider him a harmless eccentric. He gave some potion to people. One went crazy on the ward and died before morning, the other is coming around. His drugs are formulated by Chinese scientists in Red China. A French doctor has said they use lots of arsenic, lead, and mercury. These patients were probably suffering heavy metal poisoning.

Some Vietnamese, I'm told, are superstitious. Never leave home on the 7th or return on a date with a number three. Bad luck if the first person you see is a woman. Men won't leave their houses and will watch out the window to sight a man and then will step out the door and look at him.

It's a show-stopper to see a Montagnard with loincloth and spear come in and speak in his guttural dialect and then, when you ask, "Parley-vous Francais?" he comes back with, "Oui, Monsier," and continues in beautiful French.

I can take sufficient history to make a diagnosis, write orders, and give patients simple instructions in Vietnamese. I feel less self-conscious speaking sing-songy. They don't laugh.

I'm sending a snapshot of me at my desk in the clinic. That little girl had sores all over her body. Her father took her home after only one day in the hospital. We never heard from them again.

Bill Baxley received a note from one of his nurses, written in English, saying, "I want to make children for you." It turns out that the VN word for "make" is "lam" which also means to serve as or to act as. What the message means is, "I want to act as your child." It is a VN custom for a person to adopt a respected person as a surrogate parent.

7

Disconnects and Flash-Points

When Doing Your Job and Not Doing Your Job
Is the Same Thing

Is our relationship with time to be one of harmony or one of mastery? Is time to be our silent companion or part of our armamentarium? Are we to be its boss or its servant? Or slave? Usually, when two opposing views of the significance of time clash between people, we find a way to smile and joke about it. We joke about "African" time, "Caribbean" time, and "Asian" time when we encounter this mismatch. But sometimes we don't feel like joking. At those times the real issue isn't about time at all. It's about something else, and we know what that something else is: control. (Then, again, sometimes we only think we know.)

The attitude of the advisors here, and now our attitude, is that the Vietnamese are lazy, insensitive, and want Americans to do all their work. There is already enough money and goods sent to this country to make great advances. Before any more comes over I would recommend the Vietnamese start helping themselves. There is a pacification program going on in the Central Highlands. It's to win over the Montagnards. We're now in the heart of Montagnard country. There were no ethnic Vietnamese here 20 years ago. Now the Vietnamese are here. Although in the minority the ethnic Vietnamese discriminate against these people in the hospital, the schools, and in jobs. The U.S. sends out psychological warfare teams to win over the villages. Then the VN soldiers come and loot. Soon I'll be leaving on mobile trips. We'd like a Vietnamese doctor or nurse to accompany us but they refuse.

System Dysfunction vs "Streetwise":
Two Views from a Runaway Train

What we now call "system dysfunction" and habits of corruption, another might consider merely being streetwise. What we perceive as the wrong priorities might, considering the circumstances, be considered by someone else, "looking out for number one." Sometimes, when you are doing the best you can with what you have in unpredictable and dangerous times and anyone can find fault, you grow thick skin. The real question to ask yourself is what you would do were you in his or her shoes. (The joke, that you shouldn't complain about somebody else until you've walked a mile in his shoes, because, that way, you'd be a mile away and, besides, you'd have his shoes, is reassuringly funny because it masks a painfully sharp point. Being in another's shoes can backfire and be unnerving. You might find yourself feeling or doing exactly the same as that other. So one laughs at that joke.) I complained because Dr. Niem wasn't compelling others to behave properly and I ridiculed my superiors for setting impossible parameters for our mission, whereas if I'd thought about it and really put myself in the others' shoes, I'd have seen that the other was in the same pickle I was. We were all on the same runaway train and no one was in control and the train could not be stopped and it was no one's fault. Relief would only come if all of us, together and with the same sincerity and trust and at the same moment in time, made it stop. Not likely. China, Russia, France, Vietnam, America; none of these countries' leaders, I believe, wanted to continue down this track, this interminable stalemate. But we were all helpless, all puppets, not of one or another of us, but of this mindless runaway train. That's the scary, unnerving part. You can't blame a train.

I met with Dr. Niem and told him some of the facts of his hospital. He was surprised and very upset. He explained the background of the problem. What it amounts to is his staff feel they are doctors. The system doesn't have any program of supervision or control; everybody is autonomous. And, they are all appointed. Dr. Niem can't fire them. They keep erratic working hours, sit behind their desks all day, do no nursing or bedside care. They kick patients out arbitrarily. It's terrible. And now we've just received a new directive about MILPHAP activities, direct from the people who have no idea what's going on here. We are not to take control of any hospital facility but work with our counterparts. We are to train the VN staff. We are not to indicate, in any way, that we know more or that our way is better than theirs. We are to do what the medicine chief asks. But Dr. Niem asked us to send a mobile team to neighboring Quang Duc province where a plague epidemic was reported while at the same time we were directed not to work outside Dar Lac Province, meaning we should not go microbe hunting in Quang Duc Province. Likewise, we are to provide support for the Advisory Team when requested but the Advisory Team here wants me to go with the Psychological Warfare Team to villages, something we're not to do. We are not to go on MEDCAP missions where the Psy-Warfare Team operates. We get these conflicting directives from our higher-ups.

Looking back, I blame the notion that Communism was "evil" for much of our predicament. Bad, yes; deceptive and harmful, yes. But evil, no. If evil, then you can't and don't negotiate with it. You don't compromise. So we were all, Dr. Niem, MILPHAP, our supervisors, his, on this runaway train. This was our invisible puppeteer. Our leaders who convinced us all that Communism was evil were trapped by that rhetoric and we were, too. The children were taunting one another, "You're a traitor!" "No, you are!" "You're a puppet!" "No, you are!" Just like *their* parents did. (And I'm not talking here about surrendering. I'm talking about a cease-fire and talking. Just that. If you're talking, you're not killing. Surely all sides could have agreed to stop the killing and talk instead. That would have been a good thing, yes?)

Status Report, Course Correction and "General Quarters!"

Malaria, skin diseases, anemia, and diarrhea were treatable. Typhoid fever was treatable if caught early, at least before intestinal perforation. Cholera and plague were curable if treated early. Advanced goiter and cleft palate were correctable with surgery.

People died of diphtheria and tetanus because of delayed treatment. Abscesses and burns were treatable. I treated 50 patients one busy day.

Most intestinal parasites (hookworm, ascariasis, pinworm) were curable, as was scabies. Tuberculosis (nearly everyone over 15 tested positive) and leprosy (estimated at 5,000 cases) were not.

Nutritional edema, nephrosis and meningitis could be treatable. Advanced trachoma and glaucoma were not, nor was blackwater fever, a complication of malaria. Cases of malaria refractory to chloroquine might be treatable with the new anti-malarial drug recently investigated at the 3rd Field Hospital.

We pick up needles, gauze, and zephiran from the 155th Aviation Company and buy Dial soap at the MACV PX. We pass them on to my counterparts.

My medical school alumni association and friends send supplies, including griseofulvin, that cures disfiguring ringworm.

Epilepsy, eczema, asthma and congestive heart failure were treatable when we received supplies mailed us from sympathetic friends in the United States but we were subsequently warned by State Department notice to stop soliciting and using supplies from outside channels.

Most of the medications available through the ministry of health channels are of Asian manufacture and in short supply. MILPHAP, of course, is enjoined from going outside these channels for supplies as that would undermine the political objective of our mission.

The day before that big rain I gathered my canteen, ammunition, medical kit, etc. and hooked them to my web belt and took my helmet and poncho and laid it all by my bed. Just on impulse. That night we were awakened by small arms fire coming into the compound. I didn't hear the "General Quarters" siren. My roommate had to shake me. In the darkness I slipped my bare feet into my boots dressed, grabbed my weapon and gear and ran to my station. Bill, next door, didn't even dress. He just threw his weapon on over his undies and ran into the rain. The All Clear came half-hour later. No one knows what really happened. Who fired the shots? Where were they? The only casualty was an infantry captain who stubbed his toe running in the dark. Now, when I go on trips or drives, I go armed.

Western Medicine Meets Chinese Medicine: I Pass a Delicate Test

My only other house-call came yesterday. The province chief, a Paris-educated general in the army, asked for a doctor. This is unusual because he always seeks out the Chinese medicine man before consulting an American medic. He never goes to Vietnamese doctors. I examined him in his office. Of course, I noticed all the marks of the Chinese "witch doctor." Diagnosis: common cold. I gave him some samples I'd brought from home of a new 8-hour aspirin tablet (so he'd not recognize it) and some anti-histamine, and told him he'd be sick the rest of the week. If I can't cure him at least I can predict his course. He served me drinks afterwards in his home. He was impressed when I wrote out directions in Vietnamese.

Unlike my abrupt exposure to the complexity of ethnic Vietnamese identity, slower was my introduction to the complexity of the local approaches to illness. Practiced side by side with Western medicine were a variety of other approaches such as the Sino-Vietnamese practice (the so-called Chinese medicine whereby, for example, a Western-educated professional would seek hot suction cups along with antibiotic treatment).

These Sino-Vietnamese practitioners that I called "witch doctors" of "Chinese treatment" let blood, pinched, and used suction cups along with administering medicine they mixed themselves. One advantage to seeing such a "doctor" was his ready availability, his inexpensive cost, and his explanations linking diagnosis to treatment that were clear and logical in terms of traditional Vietnamese thinking. Also there were the Vietnamese sorcerers who knew how to make the amulets and intone the formulas against evil spirits. And, finally, the Montagnard way. This last centered on animal sacrifice with ritual prayers (e.g., a Rhade would sacrifice an animal and chant prayers). At the same time they, too, would accept aspirin to bring down a fever. The important point was that most of these alternative methods were nontoxic, like some of the so-called Chinese medicines prepared in pharmacies in Cholon, Saigon and Tan An. But delaying effective Western treatment regularly proved fatal.

We were led to believe we were filling a void in healthcare. There wasn't a void. There was, instead, a mixture of traditional practices already present. We were simply providing an alternative, although, at times, it felt like we were there to discredit, if not eradicate, those familiar and trusted alternatives. So often I wanted to discredit them. I wanted to do good so badly.

Emotional Distress Across Cultures: A Correct Reading of Signs

I came early to afternoon clinic. Hank's interpreter, Nguyen Chinh, hurried in saying someone next door was unconscious, had taken an overdose of phenobarbital. I went to the examining table and saw a young Vietnamese man lying quite out of it with a tremor of his eyelids. I raised his hands and legs and they dropped down limply. A crowd gathered around including the youth's uncle. I tapped the patient's knees and ankles as if to assess reflexes and the people "ahh'd" as the limbs responded, but I did it because I was suspicious of those fluttering eyelids and didn't want to be obvious. I raised the patient's arm over his face and let it drop, deliberately aiming to drop it on the patients nose. (I'd position my other hand to protect his face, something he couldn't have known.) It repeatedly missed his nose; his arm would fall limply all over the place but never onto his face. I asked some questions and learned that the boy had had an argument with his uncle and had left very angry. I told Hoan to tell the uncle in a loud voice that the boy would be all right. He would wake up in 20 minutes. I returned to my desk.

Hoan, troubled by the drama, asked me, "Don't you think he took that overdose of phenobarbital?" I told him we'd know in 20 minutes.

Twenty minutes later the boy "miraculously" came to. He acted groggy for several minutes, then left in the care of his doting uncle. Emotional illnesses do cross culture barriers.

Also Worthy of Note

I go to meet Dr. Niem tomorrow. Stan becomes too impatient and angry so I'll be spokesman. Two people in one of the districts died from Chinese medicine man treatment. The five children, orphans now, were sent here for observation. The clerk refused them admission. We insisted and he agreed but only if they pay in advance. We blew up. No one else has to pay in advance. We said we'd pay the bill ourselves. They were admitted to Stan's ward. But staff there won't feed them. It also turns out that Stan's nurse was caught evicting two Montagnards to make room for some Vietnamese. This is crazy.

Dr. Niem held a special meeting with his staff. He told them they were lazy and to shape up.

The USAID man led me into the village and down a gully to a stream with pretty terraced rice paddies. A handsome young Rhade man lay on the opposite bank, in the water and under the reeds. Downstream near-naked women and girls had stopped pounding dirty laundry against the rocks to watch, apprehensive. The man had a knife. The villagers were terrified. I watched, too. The young man began singing a lament in Rhade and made frequent praying gestures. I was awed and moved. Then he got up, turned upstream, and began boxing an unseen foe. When he finally came out of the water he let me take him into custody. I took him in my jeep to a place of confinement before transfer to Saigon and psychiatric examination. This last was my first house-call. I learned the young man, whose father was French, had served several years with the Special Forces and had even created a legend for himself. Only 23 years old he rose from private to company commander and was the acknowledged "chief" of Rhade tribesmen in the Special Forces. But he was struck with what looked like schizophrenia [however, more likely, heavy metal toxicity with psychosis].

Things are quiet. One of the outposts outside town was mortared last night, no casualties reported. Each night, to harass the V.C. in the jungle outside town the artillery fires pot-shots. They fired a few rounds yesterday in the afternoon. I nearly jumped under my desk. But the patients I was seeing didn't seem to mind.

Nocturnal emissions were a not uncommon complaint, usually of young Vietnamese men who come to the clinic asking for intra-muscular camphor, as if an important out-of-balance life force must be chemically restored.

I took a jeep ride with my MACV roommate to a Montagnard village where he checked on the Popular Forces there and picked up information on Vietcong activities. It was a scenic trip, beautiful cottages and corn fields hacked out of the jungle, vine shelters over neat winding streams where women wash clothes, Montagnard longhouses on stilts with water buffalo living underneath, and curious children gathering wherever we stop. We had tea and guava in the chief's home.

Sometimes patients were brought to us too late. Sometimes there was time and we knew the diagnosis but not the treatment. Sometimes we knew the treatment but it wasn't available. Sometimes we knew the treatment, it was available, but not in a form an infant could take. Sometimes we just made the wrong diagnosis or made the right one after it was too late.

One desperate mother kept trying to force her 9 month-old infant to swallow adult-size pills. She used a spoon and water. But the child was already dead, drowned from the water forced down its lungs. I tried mouth-to-mouth and closed-chest massage but couldn't bring him back. He'd come in with diarrhea.

I'm troubled by the practice of injections of nikethamide, a powerful cerebral stimulant, as the sole treatment for typhoid fever or for high fever in a newborn or for suspected cholera. After observing more than a few deaths, I included these observations in my first monthly report along with my assessment that this is inappropriate.

I made several mobile trips and had a miserable time dispensing pills. I was unable to give the treatment the people needed.

The missionaries from the Christian Alliance Mission educated me about the particularly toxic aphrodisiacs that young Rhade men preferred when looking to seduce Christian Rhade girls. A brand sold locally was called "Japanese chewing gum." The unsuspecting girl, after a young man slipped her the drug, could end up quite delirious and crazed.

I saw 257 patients last week. There was a boy with a soft, pinkish raised rash on his elbow and slight discoloration of his ear lobe. The area was insensitive to pin prick. Leprosy. I saw end-stage glaucoma with almost total blindness. Cancer is common, and cerebral palsy.

I've been preoccupied with a sick child on the charity ward. I admitted him 10 days ago and continue to look in on him even though he's not under MILPHAP care. He is 12 years-old and very, very sick with fever, tremors, hemorrhages from his mouth and nose and a strange rash. We don't know the diagnosis. The (American) doctor covering that ward is waiting for him to die. But as long as I have tricks up my sleeve I'll continue to write new orders on him. His illness has mimicked some familiar diseases but the treatment for those hasn't brought any change. I've treated him for typhoid fever, septicemia, tetanus, and diphtheria. Now he has blood in his urine, generalized swelling, and is delirious. My latest idea was cerebral malaria even though the lab test was negative. I visit him 2–3 times daily. Stan and I have also considered poisoning or fungus; we've no way of proving either let alone treating either. If he does have malaria he'll begin to improve by tomorrow. The uncertainty, the inability to make the diagnosis, is frustrating.

Arthur Godfrey will be at the Bungalow, another USO show. I thought he was an old man by now. What is he doing out here?

There are no major campaigns around Ban Me Thuot. The monsoon rains haven't yet come down in force so no Vietcong offensive. By October they'll have lost their chance. We know there are several NVN regiments opposite us in Cambodia but they won't make a move while there are so many hours of clear sky.

Vietnamese sleep on wooden boards with only a mat. No wonder their posture is so incredible. Their backs are perfectly straight. Chronic back problems are unknown here.

MILPHAP vs. MEDCAP

During a visit to Saigon to investigate why I hadn't been paid (my checks were to be sent to my bank at home) I had the opportunity to observe a Medcap operation.

I went with a Mobile Team by jeep to a hamlet outside Saigon in Gia Dinh province. They held sick-call by the rice-paddies in the front yard of what appeared to be a home. The corpsmen took the bulk of the work, their doctor seeing selected patients. These enlisted men are trained for this and I realized our own handicap. Our team is made up primarily of privates, many who can't read a thermometer. Because they had only one interpreter I found myself translating for the corpsmen as well as consulting. Because there are so many medical facilities in Saigon these guys scrounge supplies in bulk. They are thus equipped to make these mobile trips. However they are practicing MEDCAP medicine or "tail-gate" medicine. It's a one-shot affair. There is no follow-up, no return visit, no records, no laboratory (and thus no diagnosis). It's a massive give-away exercise with four-way cold tablets being the staple "gift."

I also had the opportunity to attend rounds at the Saigon Medical School Hospital—first-rate doctors and teachers. I went on rounds, conducted in English, and it was over my head. I consulted about the case of the febrile 12-year-old boy on our charity ward. From this consultation with the chief of medicine I concluded that that boy did have typhoid fever. But as we were out of chloromycetin, he never did get the effective treatment. The day I'd left for Saigon this drug arrived and treatment was begun. Upon returning to Ban Me Thuot I learned he'd died just the same.

I also had opportunity to see how the MILPHAP Team in Saigon fared:

> First, Saigon was terribly hot, sticky, filthy, and crowded. I stayed with the MILPHAP Team there in their villa. They've two roomy villas with modern air conditioning, a live-in cook and their own movie projector but tap water isn't drinkable. On my first night I heard mortar fire. They live 1 mile from the Ton Son Nhut Air Base. Everybody raced upstairs to see the fireworks. Being so used to nightly artillery where we harass the V.C. I wasn't interested. Next day I read it was V.C. mortars. They'd hit the air-base and killed one man and wounded several others.
>
> These guys love their villa and don't want to leave Saigon even though the weather is awful, the hospital doesn't need them, and their MEDCAP-type mobile trips are worthless and even though the officers bunk with enlisted men and their morale is rock bottom. I told them about our cool weather and drinkable tap water. I realized how lucky I was to be in Ban Me Thuot. Also, because the other Army MILPHAP Team that trained with us at Fort Sam, now stationed north of Ban Me Thuot in Pleiku, has been fired upon at their dispensary several times. The doctors work with carbines on their backs. Some sleep with their boots on.

And this.

> Here is a poem by Rudyard Kipling. I found it pasted to the wall of the MACV Surgeon's Office in Saigon.

> The end of the fight is a tombstone white
> With the name of the late deceased.
> And the epitaph drear, "A fool lies here,
> Who tried to hurry the East."

An American Idiom Is Misinterpreted: Uproar Over Words

The Vietnamese military surgeon is a prima donna. Bill Baxley, the surgeon of our team, has had numerous unpleasant encounters with him. My turn came Friday. I saw a case of advanced cancer of the breast and sent the patient to this doctor for consultation. I suspected it may have been too late for surgery. On my note I wrote, "advanced carcinoma of breast, can you operate?" (i.e. can one operate or is it too late). That afternoon, with the clinic crowded with people, this doctor marched into my office, shook hands briefly and said "Bonjour, Bac-Si Climo" and then turned to my interpreter and proceeded to deliver one of the most wild-eyed, two-minute tirades I've ever witnessed. When he'd said his piece he spun around and marched out. This was better than the USO shows we get out here. I turned to Hoan who sat down, visibly shaking. "Ong noi gi?" (What did he say?) Shaken, Hoan repeated the surgeon's message. Apparently, my question, "can you operate," which I'd intended to mean, "is this operable or is she to far advanced" was interpreted as, "Are you, as a surgeon, *capable* of operating?" The rest of his message to me was too absurd and impolite to repeat here. But Hoan said he spoke "like one who had never been educated" and that his attitude "was not like a doctor's," and so on. Hoan was terribly ashamed. This petty hysteria, based on semantics (and the surgeon doesn't even speak English), directed at my interpreter, not me, and without waiting for translation or my reply or the courtesy of a private chat — this behavior from one professional man to his colleagues — is unheard of and intolerable in the States. In future I'll refer surgical patients to Da Nang sooner than have contact with this man again.

The Many Faces of Saving Face: The Incompetent Counterpart

What if your advisee, your Vietnamese counterpart, a doctor, appears incompetent? What if, to cover her incompetence, she passes the buck, dissembles, blames, and accuses? What do you do? What *should* you do?

I now see 80 people a day and treated 350 people last week. But this isn't good and it won't happen again. The more I work the less my VN counterparts at the clinic work. They continue to go home early, leaving me and dozens of waiting patients (and with the pharmacy, lab, etc. closed down). Just yesterday as I was working, my two counterparts, the VN lady doctor, sat chatting with the technician. I asked her if she would like to see some patients. She said, no. "The patients would rather see you." So I carried the entire load. But no more. From now on I'll set a limit on patients I see and refuse to work alone.

That civilian woman doctor's husband is also a doctor. He was educated in Paris and is in the VN Army assigned to Pleiku. He came home to Ban Me Thuot on 10 days leave and ended up doing his wife's work so we got to talk. He told me she was very angry at me. It turned out she was called back to the hospital late one night because a patient I had admitted to Stan Banach's ward was having pain. She tried to read my note (history, physical exam findings, diagnosis) but couldn't understand English. She didn't know what to give the patient. If she bothered to take her own history and examine him she'd know. Anyhow, I took her husband to the ward, dug out the patient's chart and showed him in black and white where I'd written on a separate sheet, and in Vietnamese, my explicit orders that the patient receive no medicine at all. The doctor was nonplussed. Then I went on to complain that his wife writes neither history, examination, nor makes a diagnosis on patients she admits. Imagine the difficulty Stan Banach has with patients she sends him without even a diagnosis.

The doctor agreed his wife was a lousy doctor. He told me how she had complained that, earlier, I had put my hands on her. I didn't remember this. But sometimes I've been known to touch the arm or shoulder of staff when drawing their attention or talking. I told him this. He said, "She is a Vietnamese woman and doesn't like to be touched. I know. I'm her husband."

He complained that, whereas I sit in a clinic and dispense all kinds of fancy medicines and use thermometers, blood pressure cuffs, etc., his wife sits with none of these, obviously appearing 2nd best compared to me. I explained to him that I'd made out a list of all my equipment and had given it to her along with the directions that she is free to use them and also use my men any way she sees fit. To date she never availed herself of the opportunity. We both agreed, his wife's personality was difficult.

Observing a MACV Combat Advisor at Work

I rode out to a Montagnard Village with my MACV roommate. He had questions about the Popular Forces there. Had they been paid? Also about the intelligence reports on Vietcong activity and weapons and ammunition these men need in defense of their village. We held impromptu conferences in cornfields, and on the steps of longhouses. We saw a Vietnamese village chief and sipped tea inside his home and ate guava. We traveled by jeep with a Rhade interpreter and I enjoyed the trip.

The village is Buon Dung. It's picturesque, neat, clean, with maybe 300 people living there. Because it was an official trip of the 33rd Advisory Team I got to wear a black beret.

It was interesting sitting in the hut with the old man who kept smiling and laughing and bustling around like a host while his wife and children peeked through the mat wall to see us, all the time discussing grenades and mortars and routes to ambush the V.C. propagandists who come there.

The Medical Report That Stirred a Hornet's Nest

When I came back from Saigon I heard that Dr. Niem was very upset. I found out why on Monday. He called a meeting.

We all had to make reports for the first monthly record. I suppose my remarks were the most lengthy. Of my many points Dr. Niem took exception to two and called the meeting. The MILPHAP officers were there along with Dr. Niem, my outpatient doctor-counterpart, Mr. Cho (the Administrative Assistant at the hospital) and, funnily enough, the military surgeon and another military doctor, the husband of my technician [I think Dr. Niem's assistant K Sor was there as well. After the war K Sor would prove a frequent contact person for USA searches for American MIAs—Missing in Action]. These were the two comments that had made such a stink:

- *There is prolific and inappropriate use of camphor, nikethamide, injectable vitamins*
- *There is shot-gun use of antibiotics without regard for diagnosis.*

Apparently I had heaped great insult on the Vietnamese doctors. As they put it, "one doctor never criticizes the treatment of another." So the issues were, (1) were my observations valid? and, (2), does a doctor have the right to criticize another? I pointed out that the statements were true. I also said that I was obliged to report to my superiors as ordered and any discussion prior to the report with the VN was out of the question because I had no meaningful rapport with the staff aside from Dr. Niem. And they'd just said they didn't want to discuss one another's treatments.

The debate raged. One of the Vietnamese doctors opened his mouth to say it wasn't right to hurt the feelings of a colleague. They try not to offend us and see what I have done to them? I turned to Dr. Niem and, very slowly and in basic English, described the behavior of the military surgeon in my clinic several weeks before. I made it appear I'd been greatly offended because they seem to understand the language of losing face. The issue was spelled out and cleared up and the other military doctor apologized for the military surgeon.

The evidence spoke for itself. My Vietnamese doctor-counterpart had admitted two patients to Stan's ward with typhoid fever and the only

*treatment given was nikethamide, a stimulant. [It aggravates the symptoms.]
Then there were two cases she admitted to isolation, presumably for either
cholera or plague, with no orders for antibiotics, and the kid with the fever
of 105 degrees, on the verge of convulsions, was given the order for a daily
ampule of nikethamide. This was not only an overdose for a 2 month old
baby but also a convulsant drug [and potentially lethal].*

*It was clear that my doctor counter-part was the chief offender to
whom my remarks applied. The doctors' combined defense of her was
remarkable in that, rather than admit she's a dud, they rallied and said I
hadn't the right to criticize. Stan finally blurted out, "If a doctor can't criticize another doctor, then who the hell can!" Lt. Brown quietly offered that
what I'd written represented but one doctor's opinion and observations. They
were welcome to refute in a counter-report.*

*I was grateful Stan had accumulated so many charts and records to
substantiate my report.*

*My second point was defended on the grounds of patient records showing
multiple antibiotics prescribed without a diagnosis. Or, if a particular diagnosis was later established by a lab report there was no change in medications.
I described the case of the boy with typhoid fever who'd died because the
over-prescribed chloramphenicol had run out.*

*It's over now. Rumor has it Dr. Niem is very unhappy he called the
meeting. So is Mr. Cho. We work hard. Our interest is good patient care.
This is obvious. Inevitably some Vietnamese look bad in comparison and
they resent this. Since then my counterparts, the technician and the civilian
doctor, have moved into another room. We Americans in the outpatient
clinic are there all by ourselves now and this is bad. As often as I can I call
the technician over to see patients of mine. I point out physical findings and
have her listen with the stethoscope, etc. My interpreter says she doesn't like
this. Patients ask for "the American doctor" now and the Vietnamese doctor
doesn't like that either.*

The peace offering:

*Saturday night the MILPHAP officers and our sergeant were invited
to Dr. Niem's home for dinner. The Vietnamese doctors came along with
the outpatient technician. It was obviously timed to offset the awful show
in his office several weeks back. My major antagonists, the military surgeon
along with the husband of my technician, were too friendly. Rubbing knees
at the coffee table was only part of it. But the Big Two, my technician and
doctor counterparts had nothing to say to me. Of course they speak no English
but they ignored me unnecessarily. I thought I saw a breakthrough when,
last week, my technician came to my desk to take the oral thermometer. (I*

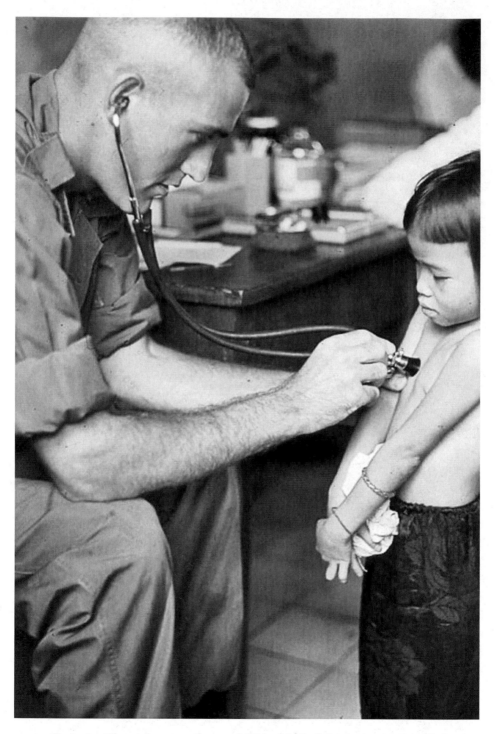

Opposite: The author examines a child by his desk in the outpatient clinic.

must remember to give her her own. She knows the supply cabinet is open to her but doesn't go near it.) She used it as a rectal thermometer.

Disconnects: A Sampler

A few big-shots visited us from Saigon this week. A colonel and a major who is our liaison officer—they spent several minutes visiting the hospital. Their visit to the outpatient clinic took as much time as it takes to shake hands. Later, in the mess hall, I attempted to bring them up to date but they seemed too interested in buying cross-bows and cameras. They flew back to Saigon after lunch so we never got to tell them that most of the people that they saw in the wards were family and friends, not patients, or that you can't simply discharge people. They stay as long as they wish. Sometimes they won't leave. I don't know the impression made on our visitors. Next we'll get another directive on how to run the show and it'll be based on this "inspection."

Our team has submitted its first report to MILPHAP HQ. We made clear that we can't initiate training programs because Dr. Niem hasn't given

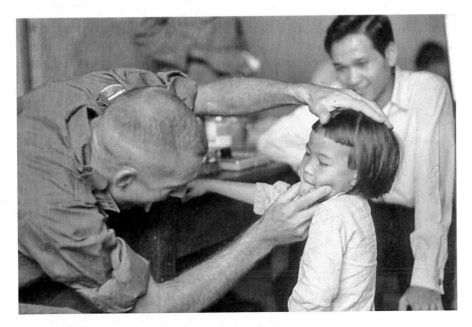

At the outpatient clinic the author examines a child; interpreter, Nguyen Hoan, on far right.

the go-ahead, and we can't make mobile trips because we haven't the supplies. Also our obligations have increased since Dr. Wheeler went home. Now we cover the Bungalow dispensary and the VN charity ward as well as treat missionaries and the 1,200 lepers out here.

Major Harris of G-4 recently spoke up at a sector meeting to denounce MILPHAP. He declared we'd better start doing some work or he'll see us out of Ban Me Thuot.

We are now informed the hospital is again out of penicillin, chloramphenicol, erythromycin, tetracycline and intravenous solutions. Yet we see them stocked on the shelves of the hospital pharmacy.

If the pharmacy doesn't have a specific medicine, the technician selects another they do have and dispenses it in the dose indicated for the original.

It's hard to believe I've been here 8 weeks. The Vietnamese have all but turned the clinic over to me. I do all the work. This is not what we had in mind. But if I work less patients will suffer. I can't attempt to train or teach them anything because Dr. Niem says to wait. It's a stalemate. I saw 80 people daily last week. I made up my mind, never again. What do I do next?

I guess I have to change. I went on two mobile trips. These were one-shot affairs like the MEDCAP missions. This was more distasteful to me than I imagined. No more. Without lab, record, or follow-up I just sat on a stool alongside a cornfield and dispensed pills.

If I wasn't so concerned about pulling this job off I'd be content. We have no supervision, no superiors here. We're responsible to none of the staff officers of the MACV Advisory Team. Our quarters are clean and sufficient. The weather is better than in most places in Vietnam.

My technician-counterpart was complaining to Hoan that the patients give her a hard time when she won't let them see me. The way it works is that when I've accumulated 40–50 patients to see I tell her, no more. I know from experience it takes both hard work and assembly line-ism to examine 40–50 before closing but she wants me to stay late until I've seen them all. She forgets that at quitting time the lab, pharmacy, and injection room lock up. I suggested she take it up with Dr. Niem. I'd stay till curfew if the rest of the staffed stayed too.

I had a good time at a wedding reception last night. It was a 10-course dinner. We ate with chopsticks. When we left we dropped in at the notorious and often off-limits International Club in BMT where the bar girls swarmed all over us drinking their thimble sized cups of "Saigon Tea" at 70 cents a shot and giggling and saying "I love you too much." Then I felt the nausea and cramps which comes with alcohol, cigarettes, and my chloroquine tablets.

Interesting news from the 155th Aviation Company outside town. A VN handyman had been observed very often dropping his work and walking *among the buildings and defense positions, pacing off distances. They grabbed him. He is the senior officer of the VC outfit in Ban Me Thuot.*

Dr. Niem asked me to make rounds on Stan's ward while he's away so I didn't attend clinic this afternoon. About 4:30 a messenger came to fetch me. It seems there was a very sick patient at the clinic. I hurried over and saw him. Several feet away, behind a desk, was the Vietnamese civilian doctor. I asked her (through the interpreter) why she didn't take the case. "I'm only taking care of public workers this afternoon," she said. My interpreter was nonplussed. After I took care of the man and was leaving Hoan said to me, "I don't understand it. She was only 3 feet away from him. But she wouldn't go look at him."

Our MILPHAP Team was feeling the strain. Word had been passed up through the sergeant to Stan, our CO, that the men had issues and wanted to talk. A meeting was arranged in the Bungalow auditorium after dinner. We officers sat on the edge of the stage, the men facing us in the front row seats. Stan began with a talk that explained the mission. It was a lengthy talk. When he finished he asked if there were questions. No hands went up. He moved to end the meeting. Sitting at his side I turned to him, interrupted him, and said I'd be interested in hearing why the men called the meeting, what they wanted to talk about. Stan drilled me with a look-to-kill. Then he turned to the men with that same look and asked, or rather dared, anyone to speak. No one moved and, with that, the meeting was over. Stan was wound so tight I dropped that bone. The men were mollified and this wasn't my issue. I was XO (executive officer) not CO (commanding officer).

Good News: A Sampler

It's September. My 4th month in-country. I came in June. Hospital conditions have improved. Outdoor privies have been built. Patients go home cured. I bought a teapot and kettle for outpatient clinic for me and my men. If the Vietnamese want to take a tea break let them buy a pot and leaves and bring their own cups. If my counter-parts won't work with me or learn from me, at least let them respect me. I'm too proud to go on making gestures of friendship. I've worked with these people 9 weeks and they still don't greet me. (I refer here to the pregnant technician and pregnant VN doctor.)

A patient I admitted with hepatitis some time ago, now cured, visited the clinic today while I was happening by and gave me a gift of two packs of Salem cigarettes. He was very grateful but also very embarrassed. It was the first token of appreciation since I began here. (I accepted his gift.)

Dr. Niem approved my taking over the charity ward inasmuch as Dr. Paulk is on administrative leave.

We're getting a first class education in tropical medicine. Malaria takes many forms and we've all been fooled. Having a lab in outpatient clinic is a tremendous asset and we've plans so expand. There is nothing like field work to learn tropical medicine. Books are a poor substitute for the real thing. Take hemoptysis (coughing up blood). Tuberculosis is the #1 cause in the West. In the East it's paragnonimus, a lung fluke. There is the malaria facies or facial look. I've heard it described but didn't realize what the professor meant until I saw it.

I see plague, tuberculosis, goiter, and rheumatoid arthritis. I see tumors, tetanus, diphtheria, rabies, and sporotrichosis. I see nephrosis, beri-beri, giardia lamblia, pernicious anemia, and malaria. I see hookworm, roundworm, pinworm, and ringworm. I see leprosy, glaucoma, pneumonia, and hepatitis. I see toxic reaction to Chinese "medicine," polio, typhoid fever and cholera; scabies, ringworm, impetigo, and eczema. Virtually everyone has a diagnosable disease.

More Man tribesmen, resettled here from North Vietnam, come in for treatment.

Having a lab in outpatient clinic now is a tremendous asset and we've plans to expand. Once we're able to culture the organisms we'll be working less in the dark. Now I am able to admit patients with a confirmed diagnosis instead of playing the odds with our meager drug supply.

The isolation ward is a ghost town. Plague and cholera are rare now. (Plague is common but in the more benign form, pestis minor.) Mumps balloon the patients face but they recover.

In the clinic the patients crowd around so close. They press me back into the corner. They surround my desk and sit at my feet. I see none of the chronic back pain, diabetes, or hypertension that was so common back at the outpatient clinic at Long Island College Hospital in Brooklyn.

Many of the illnesses are preventable. The need is intense for health reforms such as elementary sanitation, water purification, and insect and rodent control.

I made a house call on General Manh, who commands the 23rd VN Infantry Division. He had a cold.

Vietnamese Elections: Democracy in Wartime

Today, September 11, 1966, is Election Day. Americans are confined to their compounds. We've had parades, posters, peaceful demonstrations, and speeches this week and we all stayed clear. I did get a close look when a parade passed the clinic; maybe 60 people carrying signs and placards, a car with a public address system, men dancing under a dragon costume.

The Vietcong blasted the 3 bridges along the major highways leading from town. They also felled some large trees across the roads with posters threatening anyone who dared remove them. An Engineer Group was ambushed when it went to clear the road. No one knows just how many people were prevented in this way from coming to town today to vote.

Last night the artillery fired more than its usual number of rounds and some of us lost sleep. Also last night four V.C. were captured in town, part of a demolition group.

Today I covered the hospital at Dr. Niem's request (and O.K.'d by the Sector Advisor) for several hours. There was an atmosphere of holiday. The Rhade school in the field across the street was a voting place. I saw lines of people, armed RVN soldiers, and many banners. Apparently Dr. Niem wanted a doctor on duty all day in lieu of violence. My tour is over; I'm home now. I did go armed.

These elections are to select representatives who will then draw up a Constitution and protocol regarding election procedures. The election to public office will come sometime in the future. I read some of the posters which campaigned for Rhade candidates. I couldn't read the Rhade but recognized the initials, FULRO. I was surprised and pleased. This is the group which stands for an independent Montagnard state.

There is a Vietcong prisoner on Bill's surgery ward. He'd tossed a grenade into the police station several months back and killed a policeman and wounded himself. A guard is assigned to him. They sit, smoke, and chat together. The policeman wears a revolver, a simple thing to slip it out of its open holster. Sometimes they handcuff the prisoner to his bed at night. Sometimes they don't. It's like an understanding. You don't make trouble for me, I won't bother you.

A major here was kicked out and sent somewhere because he was shacking up with a local girl. He spent the night at her place during the pre-election week and was noticeably absent during a practice night-alert.

They sell an aphrodisiac in the market called "Japanese chewing gum." I don't really know what it is. There are many potions and we don't know what they are but they are toxic and have specific antidotes. The problem is that the Laotian medicines have antidotes that the VN Montagnards don't know about. Was that "schizophrenic" soldier who'd been in the river earlier a victim of some aphrodisiac? Missionaries tell me they've seen these drugs send people off the deep end. The last psychotic patient I saw was a Buddhist monk; I really don't know what to think now.

The Two-Faced Soldier

This story is about an enlisted man who felt victimized by fellow soldiers, especially officers. Every interaction left him feeling abused. Observers noted that, yes, his colleagues were abusing him, but they also noticed that his colleagues were being provoked into abusing him. This is not good in a war zone. The situation, however, didn't seriously interfere with the soldier's non-combat-related duties as part of the MACV Advisory Team, although it made things strained and worrisome for those around him. Also, it was never-ending; no one knew how to stop it. Two army medical doctors and one military psychiatrist had already examined the man and found him fit for duty. What was going on here? Was there a personality issue? Could I help?

Inasmuch as MILPHAP had assumed dispensary responsibilities for the Bungalow, as one of the temporarily covering doctors I was asked to weigh in. My conundrum was that the diagnostic investigation I proposed could possibly have an impact that, paradoxically, might render this trooper unfit for duty. But his superior officer had thrown his hands up, his people's morale was suffering, and everyone needed answers and relief. So I talked to the soldier. Rather, I listened. At first he was glib, cocky, and blaming but, after a bit, this story of his came out and our relationship adjusted accordingly.

He was abandoned by his father at age 3 and, at age 4 sent by his mother to a boarding house. His memories are of lying in bed, afraid to fall asleep, and crying to himself, "Mama, please come back." He wanted her to come to him, not be left alone. He was sure he'd been abandoned. His mother took him back after she remarried—he was age 5—and he began school. Here begins his story of being bullied, scapegoated, and in constant trouble with teachers. His cry now was, "leave me alone." He'd wander off by himself wishing to be left alone.

His adolescence was that of the loner with no friends. Kids would lay in wait for him after school. He married and his marriage ended in divorce. Now, six years later, at age 25, he is in the Army and still a private. His record shows bad reports. He's belligerent, argumentative, hostile, and negative, just as his old school record showed. Everyone he meets has something bad to say about him.

He comes to Vietnam and sees a psychiatrist. His diagnosis is "Paranoia." Here in Ban Me Thuot, Stan saw him and believed his story and his diagnosis was: Normal Male actually being persecuted. Stan passed him over to me to see what I could do. This trooper is up to his ears in trouble; the only response he elicits in people continues to be anger and hostility.

I assumed this was the same self-destructive pattern that had dogged him over the years because he told me of recurrent dreams in his life of being pursued, chased by a persistent ugly monster. My question to him was why he made people behave as they did towards him, provoking them to get angry and reject him. Why did he bait them and test them and bring out their ugly natures? (I'd told him he was that ugly monster.) Was it to get his own anger out? Or punish himself? He clearly preferred provoking anger to being ignored. In our talks I wondered: would I end up like the good parent who cares enough to discipline his child? I expect, if he makes progress as a result of these talks, he'll become sick and require transfer or hospitalization.

Several days later his friends told him what he did next. "I can't understand it," he told me. "I did such a strange thing and don't know why." In a drunken rage he tried to tear apart the dispensary (which is located, incidentally, below my personal quarters).

He came to talk to me several nights ago and began with a tirade about his persecutors. His latest crime was sleeping on guard duty and he was up for punishment. I could see the strain. That, plus the fact that he gets out of the army in one month and has no one and nothing waiting for him. Separation anxiety? A punishing parent figure is still better than nothing? I imagined this as I could see his thinking was becoming terribly rigid and any capacity for insight falling away. He began his round of accusations and I told him what they meant: "I hate them!" ("You hate your parents."), "The sergeant never wanted me!" ("Your father never wanted you.") "It's been 3 months now!" ("It's been 20 years.") His voice and his paranoia rose to screaming peak before he burst into tears. "You've been crying for 20 years," I told him. This meeting continued for 2 and a half hours and convinced me he was at risk. He had to be immediately relieved of duty and leave the compound. It was after curfew but I got permission to drive him to the dispensary at the Aviation Company for the night where I asked them to place him under observation.

My fear was that, knowing what I knew of the Nha Trang psychiatrist, he'd likely be back after a few days with the note: "No pathology found." That's what happened with the other evaluations. But I felt that the help he needed to successfully negotiate the despair, depression, and anguish that was flooding his awareness, on the one hand, and the imperative that he pull himself together with little more than those self-defeating habits as his primary tools, on the other, was too much for him to manage on his own or with me. He needed a psychiatric professional. I saw a risk of either suicide or murder. I'd pushed and he'd cracked. (This assessment was confirmed when, on the drive to the Aviation Company Dispensary, he asked to carry my carbine. I told him no.)

Gratuitous Violence: Three Stories

This first story is of an officer who felt satisfied and pleased mutilating a corpse. After killing an enemy soldier, this combat lieutenant cut an ear off the dead Vietcong soldier and brought it back to base to keep and show as a trophy. Why did he do it and why did he feel pleased with himself for doing it? Because President Johnson had made a special and secret trip to Vietnam just to fire up the troops and did so with the home-boy exhortation, "Come home with that coonskin!" So, that's what he did. He was matter-of-fact while telling me this.

... • ...

In his self-published memoir as a MACV advisor *Our War: Buon Ho, Vietnam 1966–1967* Charles Burns describes an incident when he (MACV Captain Charles Burns), Spec. 5 William Powers, the camp medic, and Y Duc, the Montagnard intelligence sergeant traveled beyond Buon Ho to where, about a kilometer away, Vietcong were reputed to be. They found none. They drank rice wine with the hamlet chief and bought some trade goods. Then:

> No one feels any pain by the time we get back to the jeep. Driving back ...
> we pass a small lake with a tiny duck waddling around the middle. Duc,
> standing up on the rear seat, yells at Powers who is driving to back up.
> Powers backs the jeep, then stops. Duc fires his carbine at the duck, miss-
> ing. Eight more shots miss. Fifty yards away, the duck waddles contemptu-
> ously around the pond ignoring the shots splashing around it. Laughing,
> no one saying anything, we all jump up, put our carbines on automatic,
> emptying the magazines, demolishing the duck. Duc taking off his harness
> and leaving his carbine, jumps into the pond and wades out grabbing the
> carcass while we cheer him on [p. 83].

... • ...

A woman attempted to cut off her thumb after bandits killed her husband, son, and brother-in-law.

Stumbling into Happy Outcomes

These were two psychiatric cases with happy outcomes. One, an American soldier I saw while covering the Bungalow dispensary, experienced relief after a conversation. The other, a traumatized child I saw at outpatient clinic, recovered despite my incorrect diagnosis.

Two more interesting psych cases. One is an alcoholic, an Air Force sergeant. who was recently passed over for promotion, his last chance as he's 55 years old. I saw he was depressed. The issue really was joined following an encounter with a lieutenant. When I told him his story back to him, only in alternative language, he began crying. We addressed his anger a bit and by the end of the hour he was back to his usual self. More, he was on his feet and animated. "Goddamn!," he'd shout, "I've been through three goddamn wars! Who else can say that!" Thus did his self-esteem recover.

In this case I saw my first case of catastrophic reaction. A 12-year old Vietnamese boy who had been in a village while it was bombed, had been in a trance ever since. He stands before me motionless, unresponsive, his gaze vacant. His arm remains extended just as I'd left it. Catatonic stupor. Post-traumatic catatonic stupor. I admitted him to Stan's ward. I paid his bill myself as his widowed mother was broke as well as hospitalized in another district.

Follow-up: On Stan's ward, routine blood tests showed falciparum malaria. A course of chloroquine and the boy recovered fully. It was cerebral malaria the whole time.

Fault Line, the Double Bind, and the "Howl"

When you are apolitical and the whole concept of politics and foreign policy is over your head — I was, in the 1960s, your average "Joe six-pack" when it came to comprehending such things — you connect the dots as best you can. This is how things added up for me. We were giving the South Vietnam government money and services throughout the 1950s with the expectation of getting something in return. And while, on the face of it, this looked like a familiar business arrangement, it wasn't. The terms were vague and the conditions flexible. The contract was so fluid and rich with layered agendas, some less hidden than others, that to someone like me, it appeared on all counts a shady business deal.

In terms of the advisory relationship that, in my simplistic view, stood in place I saw that, our president, popularly elected, was a veteran communicator and negotiator. In contrast, his opposite number, Vietnamese president Ngo Dinh Diem, was said to be an odd duck with no listening skills and a scary, retrograde agenda. But he was a serious anti–Communist and became the first president of South Vietnam (albeit in an allegedly fraudulent 1955 plebiscite). In terms of his limited interpersonal skills, his conversations with Americans, if you can believe what others said, varied somewhere between, "Hello? Hello? Are you there? You're breaking up!" (that's the American trying to communicate with him) and a monologue (him talking) that could put you to sleep.

In terms of MACV (and the MAAG advisory program that preceded it), America's relationship with Diem seemed to follow this rough outline: the French left Vietnam in 1956 and the Americans offered Diem's non–Communist South Vietnam government what had previously been given to the French, material and finances. These came with advice (not contractual obligations) on how to use and spend them. While the details of the American advisory mission evolved and were refined over the years, its essence remained unchanged. Advisors came bearing stuff with expectations on how it should be used and these expectations were unenforceable.

There is a famous Rudyard Kipling line, "A fool lies here who tried to hustle the East," which captures two issues: one of trying to get the East to move faster, to hurry up and do something you think it should do, and, two, your acting as a steamroller to make it happen. We were the fools for trying and were now dying in the effort. Curiously, our advisory "contract" had an escape clause wherein it seemed OK for one party, the Diem government, to merely pretend to meet expectations, while the other, the providers (us), we gave public face to satisfaction. That, at any rate, seemed the gist of what was happening based on reports coming back home during the 1950s when I got my call to report for duty and began reading up on the subject and noted the murmurs of satisfaction coming from Washington. So one party, Diem's family-run government, was enabled to corrupt itself and keep the money and do its own thing without initiating our requested (and financed) reforms. For the enemy, the Vietcong, this was a propaganda boon. Having endured foreign occupation and a terrible famine barely a score years earlier, many people in the countryside, the people who occupied most of the country of South Vietnam and composed the "sea" in which the Vietcong "fish" received their sustenance, were fairly easily persuaded to favor the Communists. Why? Because the Communists promised the people that, with them, they'd be left alone and would have enough to live on. What did Diem promise? Actually, he didn't seem to be listening. The other party to this deal, the United States, was meanwhile corrupting itself with the certainty that doing *anything* was doing *something* and doing *something* was *better than doing nothing*. How so? Because it was *not* an enemy we were fighting. It was Evil.

When you are fighting evil is there really an expectation that you measure outcome carefully or that documentation or data is important, or that you might need a Plan B in case Communism is not really evil, just a malevolent system of government? Naturally, there can be no negotiating. One does not negotiate, one does not compromise with evil. Since when does a Holy Crusade require careful measures of performance improvement or quality assurance? So why were we fighting in Vietnam? What was *our* propaganda pitch? We were fighting because we could and because we had to. But this was not what the Vietnamese in the countryside needed to hear let alone cared to hear. And if becoming Communist would be deleterious to them at their autonomous village level, that water was long gone under the bridge. The French had taken away their autonomy generations before. So the Vietcong offered something, a sound-bite that made sense. Diem offered nothing. Worse, he harassed the people and took things away. The insurgency was easily winning the propaganda war, winning the "hearts and minds" of the people outside the cities. (Again, these were my views.)

Which leader was really the puppet here, ours or theirs? Had that lady in the park with bread crumbs trained the squirrels to come to her? Or had the squirrels in the park trained the lady to bring bread crumbs to them? Or were they both, by that time, puppets acting under the control of some impersonal addiction or habit, a trap of their own making? If either wanted to stop, they certainly acted as if they could not stop.

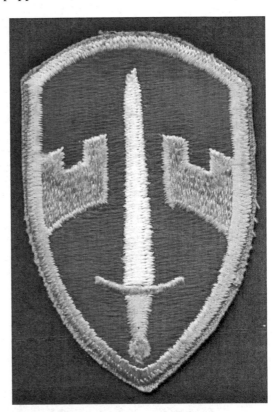

America was in just such a trap. Even if we wanted to, we couldn't stop. And the bind was a *double* bind. America was enjoined from giving our goods and our money without getting something in return. We were also unable to get that something even as we couldn't stop giving. But we couldn't walk away from the situation, either. We were in too deep. Whatever we did or didn't do we'd be risking either our integrity and honor or our peace of mind and self-respect. Or our treasure and our lives. The image of a fault line in the MACV mission was aptly, if perversely, captured in the patch we all wore on the left shoulders of

Officially, the red background is meant to represent the infiltration and oppression from beyond the embattled wall, the Great Wall of China. The opening in that wall through which the infiltration and oppression flow is here blocked by the sword representing US military aid and support. The wall is arched upwards in reference to the offensive action pushing that aggressor back.

our uniforms. It was a castle battlement spanning a red field. The battlement was interrupted in the center and, thrusting upward into this breach, was a sword. If that battlement represented our mission, then its interruption, iron- ically, could be seen as a fault line. The sword, breaking through the breach — what did that represent? For me, a sword is either something that kills or, on our patch, something that keeps the breach open so someone or something can get away. I'm good with either interpretation.

So I opted to get away. Our big buildup was underway, so it was time for American action, anyway. The advisory concept seemed to have run its course. I got out of that advisor bind, at least partially, by seeking something different. I planned to spend time out of Ban Me Thuot and in the districts regardless of V.C. A Vietnamese friend and journalist recently pointed out to me by means of a Buddhist tale that you never know what's next. Good follows bad as bad follows good so, after the bad, you wait and endure; good will find its way back to you. So, in exchange for the euphoric highs when things go great and the devastating lows when all seems lost, there is this other way, this middle way, that simply offers a way to hang in there and move on and always manage to be at peace. But I wasn't thinking this way at that time. This tale had been offered to me too late. At that time I was just thinking to flee the problem. So I asked Doctor Niem to assign me to as many mobile trips as he felt were necessary and possible. Inside I was wanting to howl, and that wasn't good. I ran instead.

Here in Ban Me Thuot there are the 23rd VN Division soldiers. They don't go out at night, no patrols on weekends, they avoid contact with the enemy. They break off operations for lunch, insist on being home by 5:00. I hear this from friends who are MACV advisors to the RVN. As for myself, I see what I see.

I don't know what they print in papers at home but out here the attitude is that Americans do the fighting; Koreans do more than their share.

We've heard rumors. FULRO says it can take over Dar Lac Province within 3 months.

Heard that, somewhere in Vietnam, a GI was drunk and was losing money at cards. He pulled out a grenade. Twelve wounded and two dead, all Americans.

MILPHAP in the Crosshairs: A Meditation on Blaming

I'll tell this story as it unfolded. Some of our officer friends began giving us discreet warnings. "You fellows better shape up. People are out to get you."

We asked a few questions and found out that a Maj. Hereford (G-4) here has been remarking around that the MILPHAP Team better start doing some work or he's going to get us "the hell out of Ban Me Thuot and into the boonies." And, if that doesn't work, we'll soon be working for G-4. He had bad-mouthed us before, publicly, during sector meetings. So, who is Major Hereford? None of us have ever met him; he's never visited the hospital. He has no authority or control over us.

Well, this unexpected attack precipitated a long-standing but never discussed issue. For all our time and work here, completely on our own and with less than meaningless "visits" from the medical director of II Corps Area and our superiors in Saigon, we've long felt that no one knows what we do. Even Dr. Niem, to my knowledge, hasn't visited the clinic. Yet, a man who has never spoken to us or visited the hospital, brings us under criticism?

Some captain friends advised us, "Well, then, tell your story" And so we did. One major made a 2-hour visit to the hospital and Stan gave him the drill. "Why haven't you told people about your work?" the visitor asked. The trouble was, we told him, no one seemed interested. Did anyone know, for example, that:

- *we run 3 of the 4 hospital wards*
- *cover minor surgery and outpatient clinic*
- *set up a complete lab with 2 technicians in outpatient clinic*
- *organized sanitary construction and had additional examining tables built along with cabinets, screens, and had given them to the hospital*
- *make MEDCAP trips complete with record keeping, labs, and follow-up*
- *take care of the missionaries, their workers and their hundreds of lepers from the Leper Colony*
- *run the Bungalow Dispensary and are responsible for the 250 MACV American Advisors here*
- *go on house-visit consultation anytime for anyone (including Gen. Minh of the RVN 23rd Division, Province Chief, USAID, etc.) whose own medical doctor had been kidnapped by the V.C. several years earlier*
- *from the start, even when supplies were non-existent, we'd agreed to send teams on Psychological-Warfare trips but these were never followed through*
- *I lost more than 3 full days making more than 6 efforts this month to recon at Lac Thien District to set up a mobile trip.*

There's more, but where does this major come off telling everyone or, anyone that we don't do work. Advisors here, by and large, sit behind desks and try to keep occupied because they can work no more than their VN counterparts. Unlike us; we've plenty of work to do with or without the VN. I guess the major felt the frustration of his inactivity and gave himself a new job, getting the MILPHAP Team

In situations where one has little control, problem-solving obliges understanding the contributors or antecedents to the predicament, and blaming comes easily. But blaming always turns out to be more about feeling better, yourself, than helping something recover or improve. Dismounting from my white horse, I'd found myself getting up on a High Horse and issuing nearly identical complaints. Major Hereford blamed MILPHAP. I blamed the Vietnamese. Yet, clearly, those "elephants in the room" were American as well as Vietnamese.

Americans keep patting the Vietnamese on the back, telling them how wonderful they are, how deserving they are, how lucky they are to live under their present administration. We give them gifts and do their work for them. But, as time goes by, they do less and less. Why grow crops here in Ban Me Thuot. It's easier to ask USAID for food. Why go out on patrols? If you wait long enough the Americans will do it. At the hospital it drives us nuts. Nurses who won't budge for you, sit on their asses all day and have the nerve to ask for stethoscopes, thermometers, cups, all of which they take home with them. Three of us doctors carry the bulk of the hospital load.

Like our War on Poverty back home (this was the late 1960s), in which the poor, the ostensible target for our concern and aid, were coming under fire from some quarters for their fault in that mess, I, too, was looking to assign blame. But the Vietnamese were just as trapped as I was. They were trying to make the best of a bad situation, same as me. They were looking to make things easy on themselves, same as me. We were all in a sort of double bind. Any way we turned we'd get hurt, and we couldn't get away. Besides, isn't everyone in a capitalistic society supposed to find the advantage and seize it? Isn't our way all about "winning?" Isn't being Number One our national mantra and "looking out for number one" its iconic slogan? So, following the market metaphor, when we are agitated and our distress reaches its tipping point, don't we act to unload those emotions? Aren't our outbursts just our way of getting spoiled stock — think of dented canned goods — off the shelves? Just like the major's spoken words at his meeting and just like mine in letters home? (And, perhaps, in an indirect way, like those gratuitous acts of violence I'd observed?)

8

Mobile Trips Into
the Countryside

A Community of Defectors: Chieu Hoi

I was agitated, and I took it out on the people nearest me and made them the carriers of the toxicity I was feeling. (I call that my "howling.") Only after a bit was I able to drop it and move on.

I took my first mobile trip today and it took me to an "Open Arms" village. It's where the Vietcong who turn themselves in go to live, often in response to fliers dropped by air over the Ho Chi Minh trail or left on a field of battle. They are promised land, medical care, and a pension. Also, refugees and their families settle here. There were 250 people at this village and over the course of two days I saw 117 V.C. defectors. The majority were suspected of having malaria. The Vietnamese Government promises medical care. Americans deliver it. I promised to see the V.C. and they were the only ones I saw. I refused to treat family, children, or friends of the V.C. They were puzzled. I didn't bother explaining.

When they asked when I'd return, why couldn't I come weekly, I told them I was not coming back. I only went out today as a favor to Capt. Shephard who is in charge of the Open Arms Program here. I had to see his promises were kept with or without VN help. I told the dispensary chief here that if they wanted further medical care to request through channels for one of the Vietnamese military doctors. There are eleven of them to our three. (I know they'll refuse. It's been tried before. The general of the 23rd VN Division has already denied these requests. But this would make clear how, from the very top, some VN leaders don't care about the people.) I could go

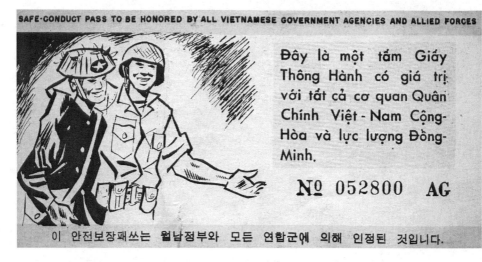

SAFE-CONDUCT PASS TO BE HONORED BY ALL VIETNAMESE GOVERNMENT AGENCIES AND ALLIED FORCES

Đây là một tấm Giấy Thông Hành có giá trị với tất cả cơ quan Quân Chính Việt - Nam Cộng - Hòa và lực lượng Đồng - Minh.

№ 052800   AG

이 안전보장패쓰는 월남정부와 모든 연합군에 의해 인정된 것입니다.

One side of a safe-conduct pass dropped in fields after battles or by air over trails to encourage Vietcong defection. By 1967 there were 75,000 defections recorded, the high numbers reached once misspellings and unintended offensive statements were eliminated, families protected from reprisal, and US forces reliably honoring these passes.

on mobile trips like this all year and I defy anyone to suggest that this American contribution rallies people to their Vietnamese government.

American policy to build this nation seems based on a premise of gift-giving. We approach their bellies with food, their jobs with tools; we reach everything but their minds. The mental set we seem to create is that this is a world of getting without giving. We reward this. It seems the less they do the more we do. The North pulls themselves up, but we pull the South up. When we leave, the structure will collapse. In a small way our experience at the hospital mirrors this. On the surface the clinic is a showpiece. The statistics show more people being treated and from farther and farther out in the province. There are more cures and fewer deaths. But the key to these statistics lies in the day-to-day and face-to-face life at the scene. I'm convinced that, ultimately, the Asian problems will be settled by Asians.

Making New Connections:
Buon Le "B," Recon at Lac Thien, and the Peanut Farmer

Bill and I, with Pfcs. Harris and Davis, took a mobile team to Buon Le "B" where we'd had rice wine last week. It was fun and we saw quite a few patients. We compiled records and arranged lab tests and follow-up visits at outpatient clinic. It was worthwhile.

Work at the hospital improves. Doctor Niem arranged for a Vietnamese team of three health workers to go to Lac Thien with me for an immunization program. This is the first genuine combined operation, genuine teamwork. This cooperation came unexpectedly. Lac Thien will be my real chance to carry out a blue ribbon mission. I see no problems. I've selected my team on the basis of performance so far. These are specialists in lab, minor surgery, etc. We know the diseases here and the capabilities of the VN health service. The Lac Thien district infirmary chief speaks English and welcomes our mobile team. He'll place us according to their needs. We'll show the villagers that American-Vietnamese teamwork is here and is here to help them. Their government wants them to come for treatment. And the local hamlet aid stations are just a chopper flight from definitive hospital care.

Last Monday I hitched a ride on a forward observation plane, a tiny L-19 ship with one extra seat behind the pilot. It carries rockets under each wing and the inside is full of smoke grenades to mark positions. What a pleasant trip. Up high we could see Cambodia. Flying low along valley

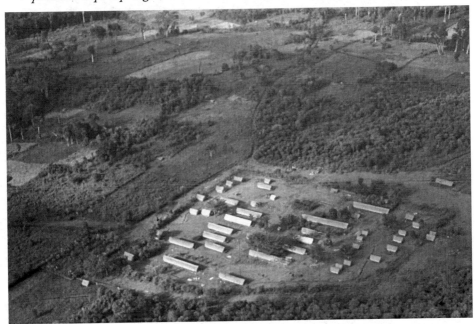

A Rhade hamlet of longhouses with fields under cultivation; e.g., sweet potatoes, corn, tobacco, cotton, and rice. Note the absence of chimneys. Cooking was done directly on the floor, the smoke intended to both preserve the structures and repel insects.

floors I saw miles of rubber and coffee plantations, mountain jungle, and neat Montagnard villages set among their cultivated fields.

The side windows were open and, with the noise, I could talk with the pilot only via the radio sets in the huge helmet. All the time I'm admiring the view and seeing nothing but rivers and jungle the pilot is writing on his windshield, "canoe hidden in reeds, 3–4 men" or "concealed tree house with 2 men" and marking the coordinates.

Suddenly, over a ridge of jungle, I saw a huge plain stretched out with a large, beautiful lake. Montagnard villages were scattered around it. There was a Special Forces camp. This was Lac Thien. The pilot landed and let me off there and I spent a day arranging for a later mobile trip. The L-19 returned and took me home. Ours was the only observation plane that day which didn't have bullet holes from ground fire. I remembered to take along and sit on my armored vest. On Tuesday I'll go out with 4 men and stay 2–4 weeks. We'll live in bunkers at the camp.

Yesterday I flew by helicopter to Buon Ho district. It consisted of some Montagnard villages around a fortified hilltop compound with the most elaborate trench and underground bunker system and 2 artillery pieces. These were manned by Regional-Popular Forces, mostly Rhade tribesmen with their bracelets, curved pipes, filed front teeth, walking barefoot, and carrying their chickens off the ends of Browning Automatic Rifles or other machine guns. I wanted to arrange for a mobile trip there after Lac Thien.

This time Bill and I and Hoan took a jeep ride to a Rhade village, population 500. We had planned to fly out to a more distant location but the USAID helicopter was held up in Pleiku and never got to Ban Me Thuot. A small boy took us for a walk into a ravine where there was an artificial pond. Nearby an old gentleman sat on the hillside with his wife under a lean-to hut. He got up and came over to greet us. He showed us the peanuts he was growing. Children laughed as we ungracefully walked the long, single-file foot bridge (no hand rails). We chatted a while and he invited us to his "other" house. He was chief of the village. We never got there. In one of the longhouses a party was in progress and we were invited in.

It was our first time inside one of these longhouses. We made ourselves comfortable and listened to young men playing music, beating on gongs of different sizes in a steady but patternless rhythm. Their "magic" man sat rocking and murmuring before a spread of many foods including a young pig roasted whole and sectioned like a loaf of bread. All the women and children were at the distant half of the room sitting in a semicircle, watching.

We saw an old man with an abscess on the back of his neck being treated by their medicine-lady who blew in his ears, cut his scalp with broken glass, and rubbed his abdomen and thighs with rolled leaves.

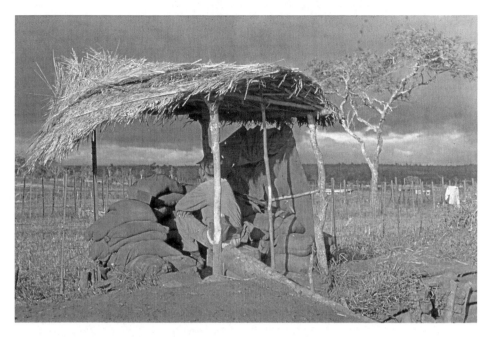

RF-PF soldier at his station at Buon Ho.

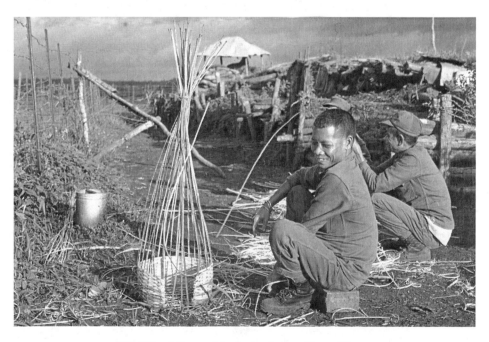

RF-PF soldiers with down time at Buon Ho.

Then Bill and I sat on logs and drank rice wine out of huge urns with a very long reed straw. When it came time to leave we asked the chief if he'd like us to hold a sick call some day. He agreed. Next Friday Bill and I will return and treat the people.

Discordance and Other Notes

This isn't a People's War, it's the Red Party's War. The masses don't willingly support the Vietcong. The V.C. control people through coercion and terror because when they don't produce the people stop believing them. To support the government there must be not only "pacification" or security, but also social reform, civic action. The government in Saigon, however, seems to remain a distant, unfriendly clique.

The more I read about Vietnam the more perplexing its problems seem. But it is a good lesson in Communism. The way I've worked it out, the Communist party is a clique of men who operate a political machine with a semi-democratic internal structure. Although a minority this clique presumes to speak for the people. Here is the big lie, the big deception. There is no debate at this level. The Party dictates what the people want and need. It is their mouthpiece but not in the sense that it listens and hears them first and then relays their word. The "will of the people" is dictated to them, forced on them. To keep it going there must be wholesale brainwashing and to channel any dissension there must be a scapegoat. They insist that the people in the South enthusiastically support them and it's the American imperialists who are interfering, imposing tyranny. We now oppose all this with arms and with "counter-insurgency" measures like our MILPHAP mission.

A friend here tells me that if V.C. are spotted in a village that village is zapped with artillery totally. Americans, I'm told, spend a lot of man-hours and nervous energy covering up this touchy topic, civilian casualties.

The other day I had my first death in outpatient clinic. While the man was waiting to be transferred to the ward he suddenly stopped breathing. We rushed around, tried to resuscitate him with intracardiac epinephrine, resuscitation bag—I injured four of his ribs trying to keep his heart pumping. Later, his wife was called from home and came to me crying. Someone must have told her about our efforts because she thanked me for trying to save him.

My former roommate at the Bungalow (I've since been moved to a double with Bill Baxley), a MACV lieutenant, is up for a Silver Star Medal for his part in an operation two days ago. It seems he wiped out a machine gun nest and 3 V.C. with a grenade. The only other news was of a reported RVN operation which ambushed some water buffalos.

Lieutenant Colonel Monroe of the MACV Advisory Team, our counterpart to General Humphreys, assures us that things have improved significantly since our arrival. Since October 1966 MILPHAP has been running three of the four hospital wards and been responsible for all minor surgery. In an average month there might be 130 inpatients, 275 outpatient visits, 10 emergency surgeries and 375 elective surgeries.

My attempts to fly to Lac Thien district to make arrangements for a mobile trip there were unsuccessful. Couldn't get a flight out. The USAID and Sector choppers weren't available and the Caribou which flies in supplies to the Special Forces camps simply wasn't going our way. All this amounted to many hours in the sun waiting at the airfield. I'm pleasantly tanned. People looking at my down-to-the-skin haircut no longer ask, "ringworm?"

Incident at Buon Ho

I returned to Buon Ho by helicopter, an exciting air ride with machine gunners stationed at either side. We flew low and frightened water buffalo. After landing I jumped off and shook hands with the major who came down to meet me. His first comment, "Where are the other docs and medics and all the supplies?" "I came alone," I told him. "Well, how can you treat hundreds of people alone?" I looked at him, dumbfounded. "Suppose you tell me why you think I came and then I'll tell you why I came."

The major told me he'd expected three doctors and a complete team for one gala Sick Call. He'd alerted all the villages and they'd come from miles around and those were his orders. I told him my mission was to support the existing Vietnamese facilities and at the time and place of my choosing. We'd come to stay 2–4 weeks, not one day. And I was there today merely to scout around. The major gave me a song-and-dance about losing face with the people and setting him back 5 years in American-Vietnamese relations. He forced my hand. Along with his medic, we scrounged supplies and went to a schoolhouse for the Great Show (and at the sacrifice of a full clinic day in Ban Me Thuot where I'd see and treat 50–80 really sick people from all over the province). I'd been suckered.

The day's entertainment was to "treat" hundreds of actually healthy but curious Montagnards, to colorful pills while unable to examine or question them in that dark, noisy, crowded schoolhouse which undermined my

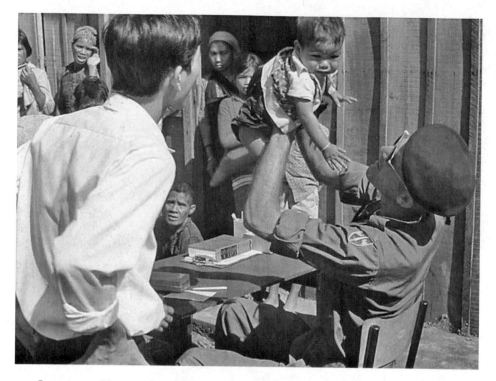

Interpreter Nguyen Hoan (left), with author, holding "sick call" at Buon Ho in the open air for the better lighting.

whole mission which was to encourage people to use their own, existing, facilities. This show belittled the VN health workers in that district and negated the capabilities of the VN district infirmary and village aid stations.

When sick call was over and my team was alone again I promptly became aware of what the major had meant when he said he went to all ends to arrange security for me. Apparently the V.C. have a bounty for American doctors. From out in the woods and fields there suddenly appeared Montagnard Rural Forces in camouflage uniforms and, during the jeep ride back to the compound, along the road and behind jungle bushes, there appeared more of those security guards.

The helicopter had been commandeered by the province chief and it looked like I would be stranded in Buon Ho but the major decided it was worth the risk to get me back to BMT. In other words to go by road which wasn't open. So we attached a small trailer to the jeep and got two Montagnards with Browning Automatic Rifles and a sergeant. and driver and, in the rain, we set out.

When we passed out of the village gate and hit the open road I chambered a round, set my carbine on automatic, and released the safety. I was very nervous. But what really turned my stools to water was when the sergeant leaned forward and shouted to me, "If we're ambushed, lay out a base of fire. We'll try to run through it." Immediately after that we struck and killed a chicken. That trip, 60 mph along Highway 14 in the rain in a jeep, was a trip I'll remember.

Back in BMT I learned that the major had set the whole thing up on his own and had lied when he said he was following orders. I typed up my report, and held a meeting with his superior, Lt. Col. Monroe and Major Byrd and they fully supported me. They informed me the major was lazy and promised it would never happen again.

Mobile Trip to Lac Thien

From my journal:

The rhythmic beating of the gongs from across the long house is hypnotic, and the effect of the obligatory cup of nampay, sipped moments earlier from one of the large communal jars, is starting to take over. I know I promised the Special Forces captain I'd be alert and sober when I returned to camp after dark. But gradually another feeling dominates: This is OK. This is what I came out here to do. I let myself forget the sick people waiting, the sick child waiting. I pass out.

I'm now settled in at the Special Forces "A" Camp in Lac Thien. When we arrived, stepped off the Caribou (supply plane), their first remark was, "This is green beret country. You'll see what we mean." (MILPHAP wears the blue beret of the Sector Team that advises Regional and Popular Forces.) The Special Forces supply us with our walkie-talkies. Montagnard security guards are called "apaches." They wear black pajamas and carry machine guns and still call the enemy, "Viet Minh." [These were also called Truong San, Montagnards who'd been recruited by the CIA and trained in company size units. Their job was security for Montagnard hamlets undergoing what was called "rural development," "new life," or "rural reconstruction." They had their own chain of command.] Meanwhile, half my team and all my equipment still sits at the airstrip outside BMT. It's three days now. We've no radio reply from home. It happened that the plane could only take 5 men on its first trip and, on the 2nd trip, the pilot filled up with cattle. Thus, my other 3 men and all our supplies got bumped.

Lac Thien is a huge valley with a large central lake. Miles in the

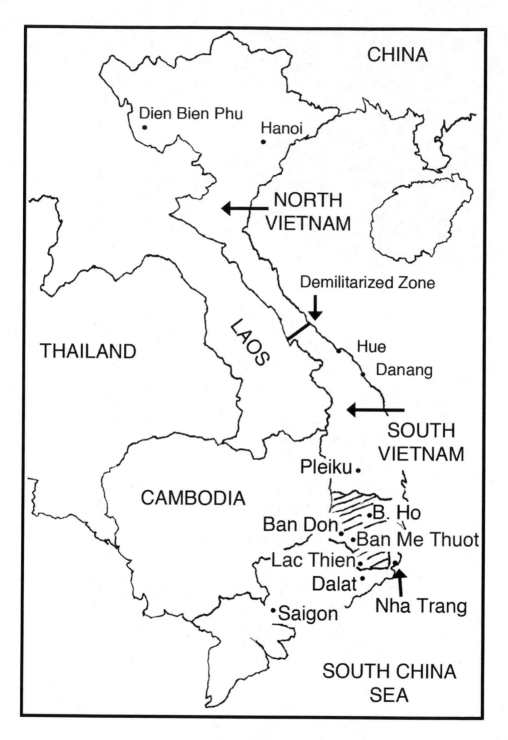

Map of Vietman.

distance you see towering mountains. Along the valley floor and set in the small foothills are many Rhade villages. All Special Forces supplies come by air. There is a tiny airstrip halfway around the lake. And what they don't land they drop out the window at 500 feet and plop here in our compound.

The Special Forces camp is a five-star shaped compound sitting on a small rise with the lake behind us and a fortified Rhade village on the other side. Stretching down the hill from the camp are rows of barbed wire and plenty of hidden claymore wines and trip flares (which cows are always setting off with a brilliant flash of orange and plenty of smoke. No harm done to the animals). It is a well-protected place with bunkers and trenches and underground tunnels, rooms, aid stations, with blockhouses at each point. In the center are huge pits with mortars. Several companies of strikers, live here with the dozen Special Forces advisors.

Since arriving I've gone with my team, including 2 Rhade from BMT, who are to immunize the people, plus the chief of the district dispensary for all the villages plus Pfcs. Guingrich, Davis, and Melberg. As a precaution the Special Forces people gave me 4 "apaches" and when I first asked what they were, they replied, "You know, assassins." At the different villages I met the chief, the rural health worker, and I inspected the hamlet aid station. We chatted about supplies and diseases and problems. Sometimes I'd be taken to see a sick or dying patient who'd refused medicine. (This is most of the people.) I'm beginning to catch on. This is the number one problem, getting people to come for treatment. The advisors back at Sector are completely wrong here. They believe that there simply aren't enough medicines or health workers out here. Not true. The problem here is getting people to come in.

I saw water buffalo slaughtered and cut up in sacrifice after a man died. We watched the funeral, the wailers, the parade of elephants. I think I understand why these people prefer a slow death with such a fantastic celebration afterwards to being in a strange hospital and dying suddenly and alone.

As we made these rounds informants came to tell of V.C. who were there in the night distributing propaganda leaflets and kidnapping young men. These villages have palisades of bamboo with sharp punji stakes set in moats, barbed wire, and small-size Popular Force soldiers with their huge weapons.

We stopped and chatted with fishermen casting nets at water's edge and boys shepherding the great ugly water buffalo wallowing in mud, and the elephants carrying wood or grazing along the trails. I sat with village chiefs in their longhouses and sipped rice wine. Shook many hands. Everywhere I told people who we were and why we came.

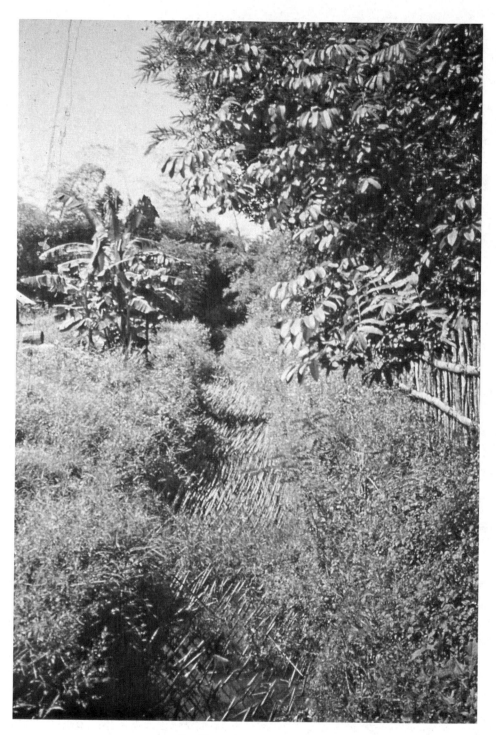

Punjie stakes set in moats.

I've dispensed with our bodyguards. One of my men is a conscientious objector and won't carry a weapon. (My Montagnard interpreter carries his machine gun.) I want to look like a medical team, not a patrol. We don't set a pattern or forecast our plans. A light plane flies over the valley with a loudspeaker announcing our presence. I carry letters of introduction from the province hospital medicine chief.

My advisors back in Sector said, "Get that district medicine chief off his ass! Set an example and treat the people!" Well, first of all, overall health is pretty good here. Second, the infirmary-dispensary is like a ghost town because no one comes. Third, the district medicine chief is poly-lingual, trained in France, and has taught rural health in Montreal with field training among Canadian Indians. He's a Rhade and has been here 34 years. He knows what he's doing. How dare they talk about him in those terms. And what's this sudden magic myth about mobile teams. People shout their mouths off about instant programs but don't know the real problems, the realities.

A Woman Hears Voices and Sick People Hide from Us

I visited a woman who has been hearing voices commanding her to run into the forest. The forest is where the evil spirits wander and bring misery and hardship. There, the voices tell her, she will die. Three times she's returned home. The Wise Lady of the village — each village has its sorcerer — said it's because of bad gods who clearly must be appeased with a blood sacrifice. When I saw this poor lady they'd butchered 2 water buffalo already. But the voices continued. We talked about this and my informants tell me that such a disease is considered a visitation by evil gods wherein ceremonies and sacrifices are the remedy. What chance have I with my medications? People blame the pills when someone treated with pills dies, which is often because they come to the aid station only when drawing their last breath. Any cure, of course, is attributed to the sacrifice or to a scalp having been ritually scratched with glass.

I haven't yet decided what we shall do here. Probably use our presence to give prestige to the health workers and gather information about the real problems so, in future, MILPHAP missions will be more appropriate. As things stand now the big shots seem to assume that just going out into the districts is good and lifesaving in and of itself. It isn't. We're here and sick people hide from us. They slip out through false walls when we make house-calls in the hamlets.

Who Goes There, Friend or Foe?

I'm busy and happy. Almost a week now. I can get so absorbed watching people weaving, building their homes, making food and rice wine, bathing in the many streams and catching fish. I play chess at the camp on an $82 carved ivory set, listen to radio Hanoi and radio Peking. The food is the best. It's early to bed and early to rise.

A light plane landed here and I spent part of the day with Dr. Lou Feinman who came for the ride. His job is running a dispensary at Nha Trang and, after I told him what I was doing out here, he turned green with envy. Other docs I've spoken to, here and in Saigon, and who treat GIs for colds and gonorrhea, all say how they wish for an assignment like mine.

More teammates and our supplies arrived late the other night. We didn't know that they landed and by the time the local Montagnard Trong San, a captain, deposited the medicine at the local infirmary-dispensary and began driving the men here, it was dark and after curfew. It was not a smart move because the strikers set out nightly ambushes with orders to shoot. Luckily, at the ambushes, they were stopped and identified themselves and allowed to continue. When they finally reached the outer gates of the camp everyone cocked weapons and turned the floodlights on them. There were lots of, "who are you?" and, "from where?" and, at last, my men walked out of the darkness scared shitless.

The Air Force flies over daily to broadcast their tape of my presence, after first buzzing the compound and announcing over their loudspeaker, "Hello down there! This is your friendly Psy Warfare pilot!." And I'd see 100 people in clinic that morning. The last day the medicine chief was picking up two patients for a med evac to Ban Me Thuot, one with half a face (Yaws? fungus?) and one with a bullet lodged in his shoulder. I selected them for their propaganda value as their villages had given them up either for dead or permanently crippled. I held sick call without an interpreter but one of the Rhade nurses spoke fluent Vietnamese so I took adequate histories and gave instructions without significant problems.

From Alfonso Rodriguez:

I remember at Buon Don Back we'd a breached presentation that we had to transfer the woman to Ban Me Thuot where the mother delivered her first baby. We had a patient, a little girl, with maggots in her scalp. We removed them and treated her. And a soldier who had a mass under his scalp [a sebaceous cyst the size of a small pear] that made him undesirable to young women. We removed it. He later came to thank us and introduced us to his future bride.

I remember going further up the road to other villages and hearing the

Rhade strikers laughing until we'd come to a certain location and they'd lock and load their weapons. So would I. I remember troops checking for land mines (and we were in a truck). I always expected to get ambushed [Alfonso Rodriguez, personal communication].

I continue to make visits to hamlets and villages, visit patients and drink the nampay at the insistence of the chief. They'd chat away while I'd drink and I couldn't understand them. I'd nod and say what little I know in Rhade and French (good-day, good-bye, how goes it, pleased to make your acquaintance, My God, very good, do you have a fever, come here, etc.) People have been marvelous in support of my mission.

The Rhade members of my team who came for the immunizations must leave on Tuesday so I've got the job of completing their mission. They only inoculated 30 people and we're set up for 12,000. The problem is that people still disappear when we arrive in some hamlets. The Special Forces are giving me a public address system with tapes of Rhade music. If this works I'll stay as long as it takes until I immunize everyone.

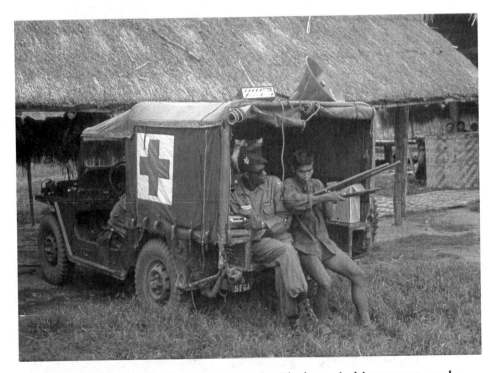

A local youth plays the ***ding nam***, a popular Rhade musical instrument, made from a gourd and bamboo pipes. Pfc. Wilbert Davis broadcasts. Hearing their music, the people would come to see and listen.

Where Local Customs and Responsibilities Clash

A village chief insisted on offering us the ceremonial rice wine after we'd inoculated his village. It was their way of expressing thanks and friendship. But there are rules. You must drink an obligatory two cups. Another two is demanded of you and you can't refuse. The idea is to have you stay there all day, to eat and sleep over and they'll provide what women you like. Different village chiefs persist to varying degrees. The other day one chief made it impossible to leave without displaying bad taste and rejection on my part.

What I'm getting at is my lab tech toppled out the sliding window and I was wasted; we all got sick. Driving back to camp late in the evening was hairy. Six elephants approached us on the trail and I kept shouting bizarre things. I vowed to refuse to accept their hospitality until I've learned how to extricate myself once we begin. Once I learn more of their customs and etiquette I'll behave properly.

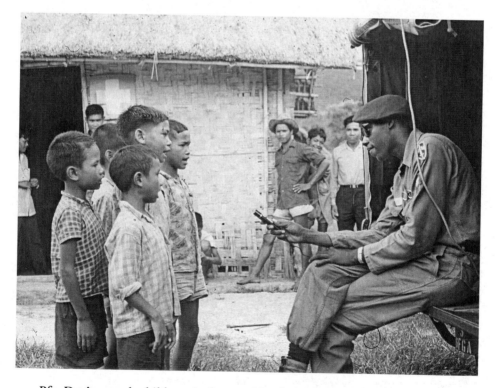

Pfc. Davis records children singing outside a hamlet aid station. (Note the faded red cross sign at the door.)

A Special Friend, the "Phantom"

Our routine. We enter hamlets and play on the loudspeaker Rhade flute and drum music recorded in another village. People gather around. The medicine chief tells them to line up for inoculations. He tells them about the infirmary-dispensary and introduces us. Afterwards we sip rice wine in the chief's hut. V.C. continue to machine gun and kidnap at night and then we come in at dawn with our own "special weapons." We're always in walkie-talkie contact with the base. If necessary we take along guards, (those Rhade and Jarai tribesmen in their black pajamas who still call the enemy "Viet Minh"). The Special Forces camp, as the others, has been adopted by an Air Force Phantom Jet wing and, occasionally, they'll fly in low in greeting. Then they'll blast our ears firing afterburners and shooting upwards spitting orange flame from their tails. One more week and our job will be done.

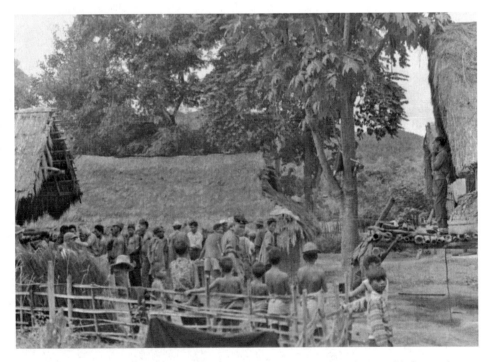

At Buon Bang (Lac Thien district), Y Rulick, dispensary medicine chief, stands (far right) on the longhouse deck and explains the process as people line up for inoculation. Speaking to the small children (center) is Pfc. Alfonso Rodriguez, wearing a beret. This day we immunized 85, were invited for rice wine, and stayed for lunch.

Our "protectors" just buzzed us at tree-top level in a series of ear-shattering passes, then made a final tight formation and wiggled wings before flying back to their airbase.

Squadron leader, Capt. (I forget his name) beat me at chess several days ago when he visited for a while. He promised to "say Hello" next time he was in the area. I enjoy that. It does a lot for morale.

Mutiny in Camp

I am sitting in the mess hall of the Special Forces camp with the Green Berets. There are many loaded shotguns. Outside, two fully armed companies of strikers wait, like us, for the outcome of the negotiations. The Vietnamese officers are tied up in another location. I conceal my knife in my boot. It is the knife my father brought back from the Pacific years before. The big issue that triggered the rebellion was food. Guys who'd been through this at other camps assure me that the Americans would, at worst, be tied up. It's the Vietnamese officers who lose their heads. We pass the time. After two to three hours of shouting and screaming it was all settled. No harm done.

After the Vietcong

About the patrol over the mountain, two companies went up as decoy. There was a firefight and four were wounded but not seriously and everybody came back O.K. Now the Air Force, RVN, and the Special Forces are planning a campaign to catch those V.C. battalions. RVN, even with a regiment, won't go into the mountain so Special Forces with their 3 companies probably will get the job. They'll set up a blocking force and then aerial bombardment will aim at driving the V.C. into the big hammer of dug-in infantry. They invited me to go along, expecting casualties. I declined. "Boom-boom," as they refer to it, begins in two days.

Right now everyone is preoccupied with the operation in progress. It's those 2 V.C. battalions over the mountain. Capt. Jackson went out with 2 companies. A howitzer was brought into camp to lay fire over the ridge. Bombers and VN infantry came in by helicopter. Dead and wounded are minimal. I had the privilege of looking at captured stuff. This one Vietcong was apparently a medic. He had plenty of drugs in his kit and also bags of letters. The medicines are all French and the captured weapons American. We pass it on to intelligence.

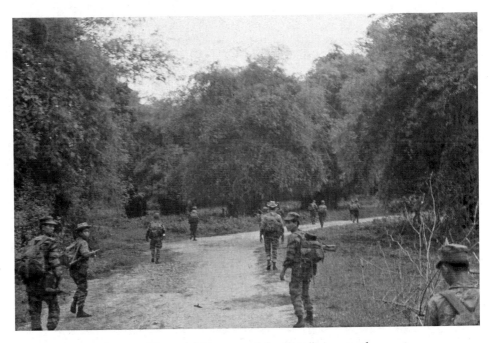

Special Forces Montagnard "strikers" on patrol

With our truck and patients we paused at the tiny airstrip to watch a caribou plane come in with supplies. He landed awkwardly tilted from wheel to wheel, ran off the runway into the brush, then, as he floundered ahead towards some stockpiled tires the pilot gunned his engines and took off again. Second time around, a neat landing. People take all this in stride.

The reason why the V.C. are able to enter villages and kidnap people is the Popular Forces guard becomes frightened. If they fight the V.C. then nobody would dare go to work in the fields the next day. They fear reprisal. Only occasionally do the RF-PFs fire back and keep the V.C. out. It's a way of life and they make these small compromises to survive.

About the Vietnamese Army, on the way back after that operation I described, the Special Forces followed the RVN infantry. They picked up ammunition, rockets, etc. that those soldiers discarded because they were so heavy. Reports are made about this, of course. I later asked my friend, an advisor to RVN, about this and he poo-poo'd it saying the amount of ammo tossed by the roadside was negligible. Nonetheless, it only takes one bullet to kill one American and the V.C. weapons that I saw were all American made.

The V.C. propaganda leaflets are telling the people that they've become lackeys of American imperialists and interventionists. They urge them to kick us out.

The Vietcong also sought to discredit MILPHAP by telling the people that the medications we distributed cause diseases. Some V.C. pamphlets even showed images of medication pills with tiny fish-hooks inside.

Sick Call and Home Visits

We hold sick call mornings in the Lac Thien district dispensary. The building is a single floor with 9 in-patient beds. It's run by Y Tang Rulick (Rhade names are gender neutral, the "Y" indicates male; "H," female) who has neither college nor medical school education. He took a 3-year course which makes him equivalent to a sophisticated nurse. In Canada he learned rural medicine; immunization, sanitary control, etc. Under him at the dispensary are 2 national nurses (like practical nurses), one malaria worker and one midwife. I am the only physician in the district.

The design of the district infirmary-dispensary, to which all constructions conform, is incredibly inefficient. It ignores the realities not only of patient load but also customs of families living in. Y Rulick, says that the more Montagnards become exposed to Western culture the greater incidence of mental symptoms. For myself and my presence here, I've tried to defer to the Vietnamese health workers and give them prestige since they'll be carrying the load when I leave. I assign my men "assistant" type roles.

The aid stations in the hamlets are grass and bamboo huts stocked with piperazine for ascariasis, a round worm intestinal parasite, chloroqine for malaria, iron tablets for anemia, and aspirin for fever. The rural health workers who run the aid stations as often as not wears loin cloth and Montagnard earrings. His training consists of a 3-week course in Ban Me Thuot.

How long does the spirit of the deceased haunt the hospital before it becomes safe for others to go there? What are the natural medicines used? What are the values and attitudes on pain, age, infirmity and death? Why does the Montagnard vocabulary seem so sparse in terms denoting subjective symptoms? I discuss these questions with Y Rulick because he is seeking to record this sort of information and publish it. In my October report to the public health director, I recommend that funds be provided for this.

While I make rounds to the huts, seeing the sick people, my team records and plays over the loudspeaker the tribesmen singing. (Montagnards have their own music and most lyrics are original and spontaneous.) Everyone turns out. Back at the dispensary some patients I'd treated 2 weeks ago — removal of cysts and benign tumors, treating wounds festering with maggots — come now, cured and healed just to watch me. They smile and stare and occasionally ask for my picture to hang on their walls.

I finally met the district chief, a political appointee and captain in the VN Army. He isn't from this area so his loyalty to the premier is, evidently, his qualification. (They didn't seem to trust the local people to elect their own district chief.) I drove up to his headquarters, showed him my credentials and, with the district medicine chief sat. He said nothing. I babbled about the lake and people. He appeared disinterested. When it came time to take my leave he opened his mouth to speak. As I waited for the translation I mentally prepared to summarize my activities, give figures of patients treated. Do you know what he asked? Would I come back to give him a complete physical! I don't like him. I replied that anytime he visits the dispensary (like everyone else) I'll gladly attend to his needs. [I was told that he would leave his heavily guarded home only when riding inside an ancient WW I armored vehicle with a turret he's secured, that's how real was the risk of his assassination and his fear.]

We've dispensed with our armed escorts, as I mentioned. The valley is secure in the day-time. Of course, at night the V.C. still kidnap and machine-gun. At daybreak I swing in with my mobile team, gather intelligence info and play on the spot loud-speaker recordings of Rhade flute and drum music. Those who come receive anti-cholera and smallpox vaccine. I carry a walkie-talkie and my men usually carry concealed sidearms.

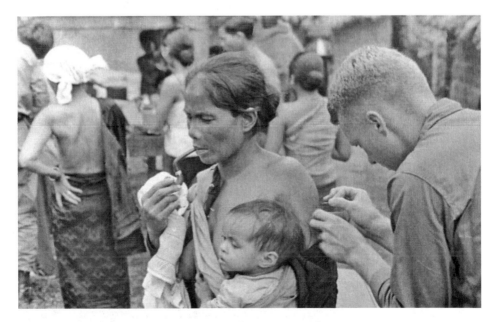

Pfc. John Guingrich giving inoculation.

At the infirmary-dispensary we've introduced some novel treatment techniques in the absence of a formal minor-surgery set-up. The Rhade nurses watch and learn. I also surprised the medicine chief when I refused to give pills to people with unimpressive complaints. And those for whom we hadn't proper medications. Instead I promised to radio home for them. (Pilots gladly deliver into my lap these medications from 500 feet.) I bring it to their villages. (Handouts that you know won't bring relief are bound to disappoint.) I'm happy with this assignment. While a big problem continues to be getting people to accept modern medicine, those that do keep us very, very busy.

The Special Forces: Lessons in Team Building

I have been much impressed with Special Forces. Their medic handles their sick bay professionally. They are cool and tough and easy to like. We talk often about young men back home, the ones you read about, looking for kicks, smoking pot, seemingly unhappy and rebellious. These fellows who serve authority, jump from planes, and live hand-to-mouth in the jungle ... same age ... have understandable disdain. As for people like me, draftees or reservists, we're the "Christmas help." At home Communism is an idea and national revolution, true and just. Out here you visit a village, completely apolitical and wanting to live in peace, and the V.C. kidnap their young men. They steal livestock (That business about their paying as they go isn't true anymore). The V.C. shoot people out of hand.

In camp the Rhade challenge the Americans to volleyball and Americans are lucky to occasionally squeeze out a victory. It's great fun with everyone attending. The GIs give them a show with much clowning and histrionics. These strikers are like teenagers anywhere, slim, muscular, very bronze, and very handsome.

Life is simple, the atmosphere is calm, my actions are fully independent, and I have help from many quarters. I've learned a lot. I don't believe I'll ever regret my experience here. Despite my disagreements with my superiors and frustrations with the Vietnamese, my time spent with Montagnards has given me a taste of enchantment.

Last night all the strikers assembled in formation at the flagpole for flag-lowering. The lieutenant, with much clowning and acrobatics, chased and led out of the line those men not wearing boots. I watched as punishment was meted out. By the time all the offenders were lined up in the center the place was in hysterics. The Lt. and his "captives" got down for pushups making

it look like such fun that the Capt. and Sgt. joined then. They did pushups with the Lt. calling numbers with plenty of faking and shouting of half-numbers, fooling everyone. At 10 he shouted, "FINI!," and everyone rose and tossed salutes. It wasn't correct military discipline, I suppose, but it was in the spirit of a boys camp. [Today we'd call it Team Building.]

Of course, behind the mountains in the distance there are two V.C. battalions and many smaller units. One reconnaissance patrol is sneaking around there now, radioing in nightly. The V.C. were spotted last night but, with the rains, they slipped away.

Also Worthy of Note

While I came to recognize the corrupt, deceitful, elitist, and intolerant nature of Communism during this period, how alien it is to the human spirit, I remained anti-war. Perhaps I'd have been pro-war if the war had been winnable as opposed to being interminably stalemated with ghastly hemorrhaging on all sides.

Since the 1920s (and the Viet Minh), if you went along with the program there was no fuss and you took orders. If you resisted there would be fighting. So we're here. I read in Esquire Magazine about a young man in an American prison protesting against the war. Funnily enough his directive to "stop this killing" was leveled only at the American soldiers. The point is that we aren't the only warriors here. Now (as opposed to my pre-war self) I know that the people [including untold numbers in the North] don't embrace Communism. They understand it as much as they understand democracy which they don't understand because they've never experienced it. [Purges, executions, and terror keep the dissidents in the North silenced.] The Communist Party lies to the people and deceives them by taking common cause with local grievances [when they have the upper hand] but resorts to horrible violence to meet genuine opposition [and terrorism when they lose that upper hand]. Communism [the idea] may be respectable but murder, theft, and tyranny are not.

From a vantage point on a UCLA campus I suppose the big picture is in better perspective. But here, seeing a Montagnard child with a bullet behind his ear ... it does things to you. All that I've described in my letters is true. My attitude has taken some hairpin curves.

The people are friendly, wave and smile. Children line up along the road when we drive by. They bow from the waist or else fold their arms and lower their eyes in a display of affection and respect.

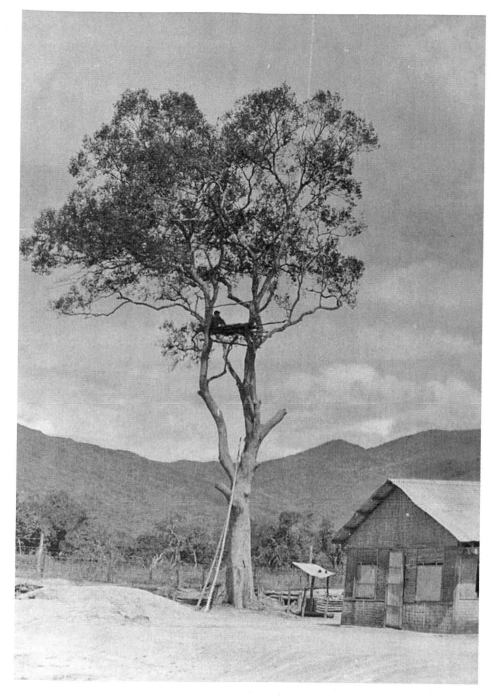

The lookout perch at the Lac Thien Special Forces camp.

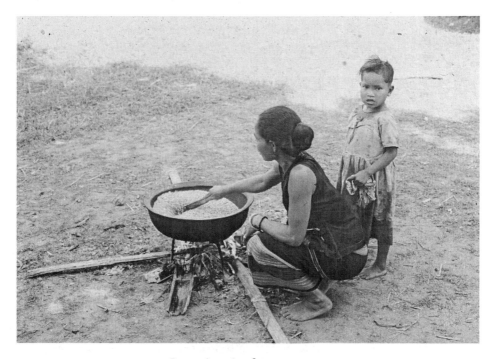

Preparing rice for nampay.

Every night patrols go out to set up ambushes. Several platoons are out now, high up in one of the mountain passes, searching for the enemy.

Sunset is a beautiful and colorful experience with the silhouette of the great tree with its platform and lookout stationed high up outlined against the brilliant orange and pinks. Its pleasant out here with sunshine and with cool lake breezes. The Chinese cook at the camp prepares tasty dishes and the meat is always fresh.

The rice wine (nampay) tastes awful in Ban Me Thuot. Like bad vinegar. Out here it's sweet, even like rosé wine. It seems they grind the rice and put into a pot over fire and add water, making a mash. Then they put it into a great urn and add water. In 3 months its ready to drink. You drink from a long reed straw which is set deep into the mash. Water is added as you are drinking so, towards the end, it looks like pale tea.

A Happy Outcome

The district health forces have adapted our techniques and resumed full responsibility. Our return Nov 1 to Ban Me Thuot will occasion no break in patient care. On top of it we were all treated to dugout canoe rides on the lake. At a final sacrifice we were presented with the traditional bracelet, and I've a crossbow and 2 V.C. booby traps to bring home. The bracelet is brass, worn on the right wrist and given as a bond of friendship, that the god of the tribesmen may watch over me.

Someone commented that MILPHAP has never been mentioned in the Army Times or any other news media. Of course, that now-disparaged MEDCAP Program (tail-gate medicine in school yards) still gets glory headlines. My attitude is, better no publicity than erroneous reporting. We were told back at Fort Sam that our mission would go unnoticed and that only our teachers at Fort Sam Field Service School and some mucky-mucks in Washington would know of our activities.

Monthly Technical Report (Abstracted), 734th Medical Detachment, October 1966

This month 132 patients received inpatient care, 277 outpatient consultation. There was 1 major operative procedures, 378 minor procedures; 10 emergency and 375 elective. There were 201 patients seen on the charity ward, 159 with definitive diagnosis; 42 were undiagnosed or left the ward without discharge. The private medicine ward treated 132 patients. Malaria was far and away the greatest medical problem including a high percentage of cases refractory to chloroquine therapy. Other diagnoses included GI infestation, upper respiratory infection, anemia, diarrheal disease, liver disease, TB, rabies, pulmonary disease (including cases of TB), liver disease including cirrhosis, hepatitis, and amebic hepatitis; also gastroenteritis, rheumatoid arthritis, cancer, trachoma, tetanus, and meningitis. An overflow from the outpatient clinic occasioned follow-up care here.

The MILPHAP mobile team made two trips to the Chieu Hoy refugee center where a total of 117 V.C. defectors were seen and/or treated. Visits are now scheduled at least once monthly plus as necessary. The majority suffer from malaria. Total number of outpatient surgeries were 405, 12 of these major surgeries. The usual cases seen in minor surgery were skin diseases such as abscesses and pyoderma. Other cases included scabies, burns, and cuts and lacerations.

At the Christian Alliance Mission there were 235 outpatient visits, approximately 50 percent of which were leprosy patients from outlying areas. (There are 5,000 leprosy patients.)

Lac Thien district dispensary provided daily sick call with lab and minor surgery set up operated by a 5-man MILPHAP Mobile Team over a 3-week period. Techniques for treating various skin disorders, HEENT disorders with removal of ungainly cysts and subcutaneous tumors, were demonstrated. An unusual generalized, pruritic yet well-defined rash with slightly elevated border was seen. It was characterized by peeling and superficial exfoliation. It was seen in all age groups. The French name for this is "dartre." Improvement in symptoms and appearance followed treatment with griseofulvin. Dx Imp. tinea imbricata.

There were three med evacs (facial ulcer, difficult labor, bullet wound) and 5 referrals to the Ban Me Thuot Hospital (hookworm, croup, rheumatic heart disease, and leprosy). Ethnic Vietnamese, although the minority group, make up a sizable portion of patients seen. It is common for tribesmen to come only when an illness is far advanced. Many discontinue treatment at early signs of improvement. A laboratory wasn't necessary as malaria is easily recognized clinically and the pharmacy is equipped to treat only ascariasis and pinworm (piperazine) anyway.

Mobile immunization teams made rounds of hamlets, working out of the aid stations there whenever possible, inoculating people against cholera and smallpox. The time, place, and actual immunization procedures were under the operational control of the medicine chief. Americans assumed the assistant role.

To bring out the villagers tape recordings were made of villagers singing, playing the flute or Ding Nam. These would be replayed over a loudspeaker. Villagers were then invited to speak or sing directly over the loudspeaker. At intervals the medicine chief would make appropriate introductions and announcements. An objective of 100 percent villagers inoculated is, at present, unrealistic because of both reluctance on their part and insufficient vaccine on ours.

The intent to demonstrate and train paramedical personnel at the Special Forces camp dispensary in techniques of stool examination wasn't possible because they have only a monocular microscope and it lacks a condenser and movable stage.

Repeated visits were made by the MILPHAP and dispensary personnel to hamlet aid stations, to meet with rural health workers and village chiefs and discuss problems of disease, supply, etc. Similar visits were made (in the company of the district and rural health workers) to the bedside of sick people where an illness was discussed and examination and treatment of the patient carried out. Prescriptions were written against the aid station drug supply whenever possible.

This MILPHAP mobile trip was publicized by a preliminary reconnais-

sance visit by the doctor, by L-19 loudspeaker flights, letters of introduction from the province medicine chief, and initial personal visits to the hamlets.

It is noted that sacrifices continue to be popular and a treatment of choice. As a result many come to the dispensary too late. Invitations to drink rice wine, dine and attend sacrifices, are generously offered.

As the 3rd week drew to a close we found ourselves doing very little work in the dispensary because our counterparts assumed total responsibility and demonstrated in this way that our departure would occasion no change in patient care.

Many hamlets lie outside a 4-mile radius of the dispensary. Our ¾ ton vehicle enabled us to make many pick-ups on the way to work. Patient loads increased to the point MILPHAP team had to ride on fenders and running board. This pick-up service ends when we leave.

My report recommended that Y Rulick be commissioned to prepare the document he'd long wanted to write on the traditional views and practices of Montagnards regarding illness, health, and healthcare.

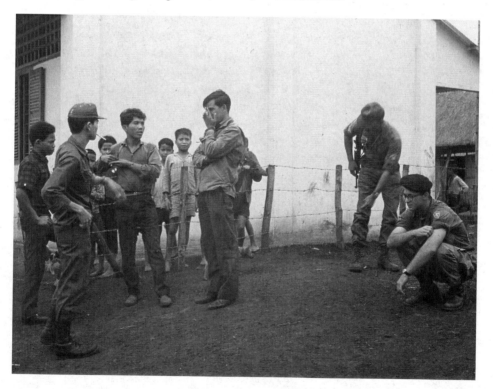

Nguyen Hoan with cap (at left); Buon Ho dispensary chief (center); and Spec. Bill Powers, MACV medic at Buon Ho (far right).

I Return to Ban Me Thuot to Rumor and Replacement: Two Things Not to Like

There are rumors of our being extended over here but McNamara's assurance that it won't happen seems honest enough. We've a MACV replacement doctor at the Bungalow. I don't like him. He picked me up at the airfield when I arrived from Lac Thien and, within five minutes, he wanted to search one of my Montagnard medics, told me my crossbow gift wasn't as nice as the new one he'd already bought in town, wanted to know why it took 3 weeks to do my job at Lac Thien without even asking what my job there was, and shat on the psych patient at the Bungalow who had consulted with him in my absence.

I've lost weight since Lac Thien. People commented. They had so little food there and what they had they shared; I tried hard to eat no more than the rest. Now, oh, God, I hear conditions at Buon Ho will be much worse.

About that new American doctor, he has a natural sneer, nervous eyes, an obnoxious manner, and an off-putting personality. His nickname is, "Howdy-Doody."

Next, Buon Ho

Outpatient clinic has literally folded. We've lost the lady doctor and technician, delivery time, and the hospital is demoralized. Like back to day one. I'm busy setting up a mobile trip to Buon Ho. In the light of lessons learned from the last visit, I've made liaison and this will be a combined operation. A Vietnamese mobile immunizing team (cholera and smallpox as before) will join us in addition to JUSPAO (Joint United States Public Affairs Office) who are in charge of Psychological Warfare and who will be contributing a troupe of actors and magician, etc. But our medical team isn't going to be just another act. We'll be operating out of the district infirmary, making home visits and providing follow-through care via the hamlet aid stations. As a civic action effort the barrage should give people something to think about.

False Alarm in An Lac

Last night I received an urgent radio message from the Special Forces camp at An Lac, a possible smallpox epidemic. This morning I flew out by

L-19 and found that their "case" was no more than a possible contact, still incubating. That means that, if they isolate the gal there there will be no epidemic. My guess is that she doesn't have smallpox. And, if she comes down with symptoms it'll be mild because she's immunized.

Bill has taken a corpsman to Buon Y Yang on a mobile trip and I'll be set to go to Buon Ho soon as he comes back. After Buon Ho maybe An Lac because they haven't anything there.

Friday Mel Allen, Stan Musial, Harmon Killebrew, and Hank Aaron with other baseball stars will visit. An Australian stripteaser will be here Saturday.

9

Lamentations and Harmonies

Enlisted Men vs Officers:
Team Bonding Outside My Comfort Zone
(Way Outside)

The large social hall at the Bungalow is full, crowded with GIs. Between 100 and 150 whistling, cheering soldiers have filled all the rows of benches. Most of the officers, like me, have (discretely) taken standing room along the sides and in the back, like teachers at a school dance. This was not a USO show; $1.50 in "script" money (issued to all GIs in Vietnam in exchange for greenbacks to keep American bills from disappearing) is the admission. On stage is a big, once beautiful, buxom, blond, strip teaser. She has just called for two volunteers. She looks over the crowd before her and the crowd before her looks to the sides and the back. As if by telepathy this crowd has decided the volunteers should be officers.

I don't know the other name they began chanting. I just heard my name. I tried smiling and shaking my head but that only egged them on. Thus bullied and shamed I made my way to the stage. Once there, myself and the other officer simply played along, "followed orders," as it were. What were her orders? With hands behind our backs we two, using only our teeth, were directed to remove the key parts of her clothing. The good news was that those parts she selected were extremely light-weight, if difficult to get our mouths around. (That was also the bad news.) There was other good news. I got the job done and received lots and lots of appreciative applause. (Maybe it was just relief it wasn't them.)

I Look a Gift Horse in the Mouth and Scare It Away

Reading what follows, keep in mind that at the Ban Me Thuot civilian hospital, there was no shortage of nurses or technicians, although it may have seemed that way because of the hours some kept and the responsibilities some ignored.

We had a surprise visit at the hospital by a very nervous and too eager American lady from Saigon. I've told you about whistle-stops people make but this was wild. Something like: "Hello. I'm Miss so-and-so from Saigon and I'm going to send you 3 American nurses." Then, turning to her escort, glancing at her watch, "Do I have another minute?" And she was getting up to leave!

Stan barely stammered, "We'll do everything possible to take care of them and work things out," but I was doing a fast boil. These gals are civilians, just out of training. That means they aren't ready to do any teaching, even if they did they'd discredit whatever teaching program already exists at the hospital, the government isn't ready to pay VN nurses for time at study so there'd never be a class, since every ward already has Vietnamese nurses and technicians, and since these American gals mustn't replace the VN, any sharing of responsibility would destroy the morale of the VN. (I could go on.)

So, as Miss X from Saigon was leaving, appearing satisfied, I tossed a bomb. "You're going to cause lots of trouble and create a mess here. It would be a serious mistake."

She had a plane to catch so she couldn't stay for discussion. The girls arrive in several weeks, if at all. Her escort, from USAID, later told us she was very upset by what I said. But the less the VN perform, some American is going to leap into the breach. The point is to develop the resources here. Even the military is planning to give RVN a 2nd chance to take on the bigger share of the fighting.

I remember the problems caused when we came. We're still trying to be accepted. Yes, American nurses will boost morale, "American" morale. Better they do something for USAID in Ban Me Thuot than the hospital for now.

I feel a sore throat coming on. The rains have begun again and nights have become very cold.

Also Worthy of Note

I am advised that people have been wondering why I wear socks with my sandals in the manner of lepers.

The average life expectancy, I read, is about 35 years. I read that half the children born don't reach their 5th birthday. 8 percent don't survive the

1st week of life. The maternal death rate is 25 times that of ours. [These statistics may have been out of date.]

Montagnards, whether going down the street or across a field, walk single-file. It must be a habit from walking trails. The men always lead carrying a weapon, the women following carrying any burdens. [This was the case even in a city, even walking a wide sidewalk.]

A trooper from the Air Force Company has asked to talk to me about his problem. He's been divorced and has remarried and his ex-wife is writing him. He needs helping deciding what to do.

Clinic has improved. I've dispensed with the lab and my teammates. Now, just me and the (new) technician; the other went to deliver her baby. The technician is hard-working and sharp. We sit side by side and go over cases together and I'm impressed with his knowledge and medical judgment. I don't worry about leaving the clinic for my mobile trips anymore.

My friend, Capt. Joe Kopec, Polish, has adopted Stan, also Polish, as a lansman. Calls him, "Stashoo." (I'm "Laurenski.") He's organized a clique including some Russians loosely clumped as the "Cossack Brotherhood." They speak their mother tongue and are now on a kick, speaking with each other in very studied Old World accent, shouting at the waitresses in Polish, etc.. To me they sound like the heavies in the movie we saw tonight, Secret Agent Fireball. I like them all but I stay by myself.

I finally read a definition of "camp" which sounds right. I once tried to explain it to Pa and got lost. I like this definition: "An amused fondness for the naive." Is camp still "in"? Is being "in" still "in"?

Some American soldiers write home decrying the conditions of the people in Vietnam, noting things like Vietnamese children growing up without ever having played a game of baseball. (Soccer is Vietnam's national sport!) Or the many kids here who don't even know what Christmas is like. (Most of the Vietnamese are Buddhist!) I know because I see clippings of hometown newspapers reporting what civic leaders are planning to do to help ameliorate these "problems."

Life here is pretty much the same. V.C. mortared the outskirts the other night. No casualties. Our patrols keep them off balance. We pick up scuttled radio sets, weapons, etc.

I want to keep on the road as much as I can. Get more done that way.

An Interpreter's Story

Since we came to Ban Me Thuot there have been 8 suicide attempts, more than half successful, all young girls, all involving romance. Stan's interpreter, Duy (Z'wi), has a younger sister, 19, who is pretty with a 4 month-old baby. During the past month she has come to clinic (or to Stan) often, complaining (e.g. her baby's urine is yellow, the baby coughs, the baby sniffles, etc.) Each time the baby is found to be healthy and happy. We'd reassure mama and offer no treatment. No second thoughts. This morning she came to Stan's ward and asked her brother for 30 nivoquine tablets for her husband (Army) to take with him on an operation. Later Duy found out there was no operation in progress. Then why did she want the pills? One of the corpsmen and Duy jumped into a jeep and went to her house. She said she threw the pills away. Suspicious. Also suspicious since she'd had a fight with her husband last night.

At noon Duy came to the Bungalow in a state of shock. I raced to the hospital to find his sister dead. Overdose, 30 nivoquine. Poor Duy went wild, screaming, kicking, beating the ground, unconsolable. Shouting, "I killed her!" As an after-note, in trying to locate the husband, it turns out he had heard the news earlier and disappeared. He was searching for a gun to kill himself.

The question is: Why is it that in conflicts of love these VN girls think first of suicide. How much is anger, how much is depression? And also, were those many visits with her baby a warning? Was it her way of asking for help? I just don't know. And Duy? He feels responsible as it was he who gave her the nivoquine. Will he be alive in the morning?

Duy, blaming himself, is going mad with grief and remorse. One of the other interpreters passed him in the market today covered with mud and dirt and asked what he was doing there. "I'm looking for my sister," he said, "but I can't find her." [Duy never fully recovered from this breakdown. After the war he taught English in Ban Me Thuot.]

The Gift Horses Return and I Leave for Buon Ho

The 3 American civilian nurses are coming to our hospital. Dr. Niem approved. It'll be a big bomb in our lap and endless trouble. Their presence will jeopardize our own tenuous rapport with our colleagues. I'll be glad to hit the road again.

Monday I'm off to Buon Ho for a 2-week mobile trip. Pfc. Harris and Sgt. Sanders and my interpreter, Hoan, will go with me. It won't be an easy trip. The MACV major who runs the compound out there thinks of us as an imposition. He wanted us to bring our own food, water, and gasoline.

But an army directive says MACV must support our mobile trips and we neither have trucks to carry these supplies nor soldiers to provide our convoy security. I was ready to call the trip off and go instead to An Lac. Finally a compromise. But if the major doesn't have supplies waiting for us when we arrive I'll make a report. Big lip service to civic action and "pacification" but Buon Ho needs this; most of that district is V.C. A VN Psychological Warfare team will be there to coordinate activities with us.

Enemy Losses vs. Allies Gained: Two Outcome Measures

We're now out of penicillin, chloroquine, and chloramphenicol, besides streptomycin. So I must go to Buon Ho with empty pockets. They've now got more than 1,000 refugees there, liberated from the Vietcong area. I'll hope for the best.

The trip to Buon Ho was a mess from the start. You remember the heartache over the planning? Who would support us with food, water, gasoline? Sub-sector people out there told us we'd have to do all this ourselves despite orders to the contrary. They said they just couldn't. After 4 weeks of aggravation I told them I was going to call the trip off. Then they said, "Come out." So I left supplies up to them. I planned to leave for Buon Ho the 28th, a Monday. Word got around and everybody knew. Fine. Because I suspected there wouldn't be a convoy going out or security forces there to protect us, at sun-up on the 27th we slipped out of Ban Me Thuot and raced along the road to Buon Ho. I didn't even tell my men until they were in the jeep and told Stan as we pulled away.

Buon Ho district is north of us. It is mostly in V.C. hands. District headquarters is a fortified compound on a red dirt hill and most of the population live in hamlets and villages around it. [The compound was about 100 yards square and housed more than 300 people, including the wives and children of the RF-PF soldiers and a half-track truck and crew. If they weren't part-time or formerly V.C., their relatives or neighbors likely were. The range of the howitzer defined the limits of district control.] There are several companies of Regional-Popular Forces there, some artillery pieces, and 5 American advisors. Those poor fellows have been stuck on that hill for 9 months and their CO is a major who worked his way up from private. He is, in my view, hypocritical, arbitrary, unpredictable, disrespectful, and insincere—a hard-assed personality.

For 2 weeks it rained and was cold and there was mud everywhere. I slept in a sleeping bag. We ate only 2 meals a day and washed out of a basin. The latrine was a hole in the ground outside the compound and out in the surrounding barbed wire. A path to the hole and a screen of bamboo by the hole gave privacy. Jungle rot got into everything. The district dispensary nearby was out of drugs. I gave the district medicine chief a program of my itinerary listing what villages I'd visit at what time on the first day. Yet everywhere we went no one was expecting us and the health workers were off in the jungle. And in some other hamlet hundreds were gathered waiting for people to immunize them, who never showed up because it wasn't on my program for that day.

The major kept baiting me for an argument. He insulted me and was generally obnoxious. I expressed my disagreements respectfully and refused to argue. Of his two men assigned to me one thought he'd tell me my job. The other was useless. A Specialist 5 William Maxwell Powers from Pennsylvania proved a helpful, reliable, and affable soldier nearing the end of his four-year enlistment, who readily contributed to our project. The cook out there, a sergeant and Bulgarian refugee from WW II, suddenly refused to feed my interpreter after the 1st week. Wouldn't give a reason.

Hoan didn't know why, either. It was as if the sergeant, like the major, neither liked nor trusted any Vietnamese. Hoan recalls:

> I still have the feeling of the time there. It was cold and a little scary, especially when we went deeper into the villages. I remember my problem with C rations but luckily there was a small place on the street I could get some food [Nguyen Hoan, personal communication].

From my journal:

There were still some pleasant moments, like watching Montagnard soldiers break up watching a Jerry Lewis movie shown outdoors in the compound, projected against the wall of a building. The soldiers on the hill actually live at their posts in mud bunkers whose "window" serves as the machine gun port. On weekends their wives, children, and sweethearts come and live with them. Otherwise, the men hated the major and the district chief hated the major. The corpsmen hated the medicine chief of the dispensary and the major hated everybody.

Most of the supplies I did bring out with me were contributions from the states. I couldn't do any teaching or training without supplies. They've got plenty of aspirin, piperazine, chloroquine, and iron. But how can I teach them to treat plague with streptomycin, dysentery with tetracyclene, pneumonia with penicillin, or skin infections with bacitracin without these drugs, ointments, or enough compresses and bandages? How I can I teach them to avoid hookworm when they have no shoes? Colds were epidemic. The refugees had sold their government given blankets for food and wouldn't eat the Bulgar Wheat USAID gave them. Didn't like the taste. (Neither did I. But I managed to force it down every morning with some C rations.) You'd tell them they'd get pneumonia if they didn't keep warm and dry, then watch them walk the 3 miles back home in chilling weather wearing nothing but a shirt. Kiddies barefoot without pants. So, colds become pneumonia and we had no antibiotics.

The Vietcong to the west still had to be dealt with. I watched Skyraiders dive bomb and Phantom jets make a frightful noise as they came to fire their rockets. Daily. One afternoon the 1st week, eating lunch back at the compound, the building began to shake and there was a terrible rumble. It kept getting closer. I thought earthquake or mortar attack. We ran outside and to the east saw black clouds of smoke. It was one of many B-52 raids we were to witness. Never saw the planes or even heard them, just the ground shaking like the world was ending and then a sound of terrible thunder.

We learned right away that the road wasn't secure. Hadn't been for weeks. V.C. were collecting taxes on the highway. So I was determined not to repeat my wild jeep ride home without armed escort. Meanwhile, in the hamlets we'd proceed in relative peace. To some far away villages we took

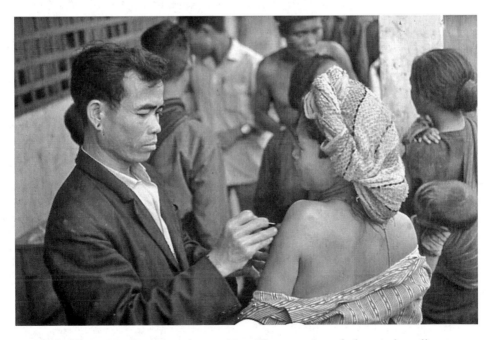

Chief of Buon Ho dispensary immunizes villagers against cholera and smallpox.

Popular Forces guards in the jeep and on the trails. I saw once again what it meant to set up security. Driving along narrow jungle tracks with the brush scraping the jeep on either side we'd pass little clearings with camouflaged soldiers or catch glimpses of machine gunners stationed behind trees, all our people. It was reassuring. We'd sit in the chief's hut after house-calls, with these people in loin cloths and blankets. The guest in one's home is a very important occasion (and that guest would be me). And, looking carefully, within reach of these Montagnards were burp guns and rifles and the new Revolutionary Development teams, teenagers volunteering like for our Peace Corps, young boys and girls trained in everything from building bamboo palisades to cooking to sanitation, dressed in the peasant black pajamas, going to live in these hamlets. These are the counterparts of the V.C. cadre who also go into villages. The VN government is getting smart, looking to beat the V.C. at their own game and at the grass roots level. These kids are full of spunk and spirit. The girls are pretty and the esprit high. They, too, were there in the village chief's hut.

So, with personalities and supplies as they were, and the rain and mud, it was miserable. But we immunized 2,000 people and treated a hell of a lot. When came time to leave the major got a report from one of his agents that a V.C. squad was seen on the southern hill with automatic rifles just where the road to Ban Me Thuot opens to uninhabited countryside. He gave us a reaction force. They rode in a truck in front of us, 15 armed soldiers, and some machine gunners in a jeep behind us. We lit out with the gas pedal down to the floor to Ban Me Thuot.

I arrived in BMT yesterday morning, unshaven and filthy, clothes worn 5 straight days. The laundry couldn't dry in the rain. And now I'm winded and my sights are on An Lac. That's our next mobile trip. But no more road runs. An Lac is too far away. We'll fly.

The American nurses haven't arrived yet. Word is they'll be here in 2–4 weeks.

Reflection: Should I have been as indignant as I was at the major's treatment of MILPHAP, his not respecting our mission? Or ought I have been embarrassed instead, at myself for not cutting him slack, for making no effort to respect *his* mission? (This became an issue for me when my friend, Spec. 5 Powers, days before his tour was up, was killed in a subsequent combat operation believed to have been against the V.C. but that, in reality, was against North Vietnamese Army regulars from the NVN 3rd battalion, 33rd regiment.) The major had truly been charged with holding the fort for the district, with the equivalent of civil guard (the RF/PFs) in a sea of Vietcong. He was out there, the first American at this location, a professional soldier who'd risen from the ranks of private (a tank driver in Germany in WW II who rose to sergeant and later received a battlefield commission at Pusan in the Korean War) and wasn't likely to be rotating out like me and mine. He was out there where everything was primitive, literally stuck in the mud. He, like me, was neither a director nor controller, just the district MACV advisor. And giving the advance notice I'd asked — assuming his counterparts even agreed — would certainly have put his American team, not just my team, at risk. (Of course none of this negates the possibility that the major was treated with such obvious disdain by his superiors as a sort of perverted payback according to some informal military merit system.) But all this became an issue only briefly. Soon after hearing of that attack on Buon Ho other trees popped up to keep me from seeing the forest. They always did.

This issue is worthy of pondering. Which would have been the better measure of success of a counterinsurgency program like ours back then, the number of V.C. killed or number of civilians seen and treated, at least well enough to recover from medical symptoms and illnesses and be grateful and pass along a good recommendation of the government side? The first method counts dead bodies of combatants. The other counts the numbers of civilians, ordinary people, the "sea" from which the V.C. drew its nourishment and without which they'd wither and die. The first had the support of tradition and was respected, the second experimental and untested. In any event, both measures would require crunching numbers by bean counters, and bean counters back then could and, I believe, sometimes did, fudge numbers to fit expectations. (Charles Burns, in his self-published memoir, *Our War: Buon Ho, Vietnam 1966–1967*, gives a close-up look at such matters at the grass-roots level. On a note of irony, Capt. Burns, a keen observer and keeper of details, makes no mention of MILPHAP in his memoir.)

More "Also Worthy of Note" Notes

Clinic has been slow for me only because my new technician is such a cracker-jack. He can handle most of the load himself. So I've been reading Rip Van Winkle in Vietnamese with Hoan's help. It's interesting because "van" is a common VN middle name, like Nguyen Van Ky. So we call Rip Van Winkle, Nguyen van Wink.

A cadaveric, ancient shriveled woman with untreated cholera (for weeks) died today. Her stools looked like rice water. She was 25 years old.

We're out of streptomycin, completely. Now plague cases are popping up, the pestis major type. In other sections of town informants report rats dying Engineers have been consulted regarding rodent control. Trying to locate flea spray. And, of course, pray for streptomycin.

The most ubiquitous medical problems on the wards still are malaria-related. Patients continue to come in only when the illness is advanced and then discontinue treatment at the early signs of improvement.

Despite being the minority group, the Vietnamese make up a sizable portion of the patients who appear for treatment. Often they displace Montagnard patients to get a hospital bed.

A patient came with a son sick with pneumonia. We admitted the boy and tried to reassure the distraught father, to no avail. Then we learned that a VN Army truck had struck and killed his other son on the way to the hospital.

Ma sent a copy of Jacques May's Siam Doctor; New Haven Public Library loaned it. This fellow was MD in Siam from 1932–1940 and wrote about it. Already I've learned something. That Chinese medicine causes kidney failure and arsenic plays a role. (I'd guessed lead.) He also wrote that Indochina's people wouldn't be ready for democracy or progress or anything new as long as most of the people carry a belly full of worms and barely 4 grams of hemoglobin.

A Department of State USAID man who'd made a whistle-stop visit last month dropped me a line. He mentioned me to Connecticut Representative Jack Bingham, who is due for a VN tour; may stop in Ban Me Thuot for a chat.

We thought the MILPHAP program would be scrapped because the army couldn't spare doctors to treat civilians. We'd heard this. But the colonel said it wasn't true. We'd have our replacements, only not one big team en masse. There'd be staggered replacements to carry on our work. This was good news.

Hoan has been my right arm. He acts as nurse, corpsman, reminds me of things to do, things left behind. He rode through the hamlets of Buon Ho District unarmed, squatted in the trailer with me, took all the risks like when we'd run an especially insecure road. I'd tell him to do and go exactly as I did if I jumped. All with good cheer and never a frown.

First World, Third World, and the American Gaffe

It has become increasingly clear that there is a communications problem between medical workers in the field and policy makers in Saigon and Washington. After 6 months I've seen much of this. Perhaps the saddest part is the denial which would favor paper reports to the facts in the field, and not see what is obvious to us here. And the visitors don't stay long enough in Ban Me Thuot to hear us explain.

It came as no surprise when I read that Ambassador Lodge, who attended the ceremony welcoming the outlawed Montagnard organization, FULRO, to the government side, refused to even sip the ceremonial rice wine. To the Montagnard, the guest in his home is an honored person. It's a very important event in his life. His hospitality is expressed in the one gift he has to offer, his rice wine. And the Ambassador "declined." To me this illustrates naivete at the highest level. Maybe he hadn't been forewarned. (Then, again, maybe he had.)

I Am Vindicated

Several hours ago we got an urgent message. Maj. Gen. Humphreys was coming here with the new VN public health minister. The general couldn't make it but the colonel came with the minister along with a Mrs. Keyes from State Department (USAID, Washington, D.C.) Stan toured the hospital with them and Bill and I joined for lunch at the province chief's. The VN military doctors were there along with other dignitaries.

First of all, they were impressed with what we've done here. They toured the VN wards and there was lots of yelling and gesturing. The VN were out in their best nurse uniforms and were quite intimidated by the public health minister. Yet they actually refused to unlock a door on their ward. (Lots of flak over this.) The minister went next to the pharmacy and took the camphor, etc. and smashed them to the floor. "GET RID OF THIS STUFF!" The two Vietnamese doctors hit the roof. The surgeon went livid and gave lip. The pharmacist and the rest were shaken up. But, feel as they might, the health minister, a political appointee, is the honcho; they dare not oppose him. The minister meant business. And, behind their backs, the colonel was flashing Stan a "thumbs up."

Later, the colonel commented about the VN medical practice, use of drugs, etc. and said, "You people must tell us about these things! We've got to know!" Stan suppressed a smile and told him, "We did make a report of it. Once." I smiled. (I made that report back in August and caused such trouble, remember?) And Pa wrote me afterwards to say I mustn't criticize the VN doctors on their practice of medicine or use of camphor. Today, the VN minister of health actually smashed all the vials of camphor that were sitting on the pharmacy shelves!

I asked Mrs. Keyes who she was and why she had come. Back in Washington she'd been getting lots of mail from drug houses, MILPHAP doctors' wives, etc. asking why there is such a shortage of supplies out here. She laid it on the line and came out here to investigate. The entourage has been, and is, in the process of making rounds of all the civilian hospitals. I told her that supplies were number one problem for us. The entourage is gone now but it was a shot in the arm. She was sweet but I don't expect anything to change. People know and are interested and want action.

Follow-up: Mrs. Keyes made her report and, subsequently, sent us a telegram. We were to stop soliciting supplies from friends in the states. This was a tough pill to swallow inasmuch as we'd pulled through so many patients because of these samples. Being hardest hit were the cardiac patients, those with congestive heart failure and asthma, the epileptics, the agitated, and those with ringworm, and eczema (to name a few). Doubly hit were the women or girls with those skin diseases that made them "not-marriageable." Griseofulvin that I'd received from the states eliminated unsightly ringworm sores on the skin of otherwise beautiful and attractive girls. Now everyone, including American medics, would go back to giving them ointments, convincing themselves (as they tried to convince me) that it was "scabies" anyway, a different condition altogether.

Reports from friends who overheard colonels and majors talking. Praising me for my work in the field.. Someone briefed today's visitors. They, too, knew of my mobile trips.

I'm making plans to fly to An Lac for several weeks on a mobile trip. It is near the Cambodian border. There are no government health services there; it isn't on the map. But there is a Special Forces camp. I'll go alone; probably spend my birthday there.

Two Laments: Both Mine

The information which informs policy-making probably makes satisfying reading in hometown papers. I believe it's written by politically-connected officials in Saigon. I know the kind of stuff they are writing because they periodically take whistle-stop forays up-country, fact-finding quickies that leave just enough time to buy some cross-bows and baskets and say hi to some big-shots and give us a few pointers and directives. Our impression is that they are misinformed, naive, and often not really interested in what's happening ... our issues. So I prefer to stay out in the field. I continue to make my monthly reports. Word has it that my work actually is known and that I've been commended in high circles for my efforts in the districts. But, as I see it, this is part of the larger process of their reading what they want to read and believing what they like and accepting a paper illusion. Then they feel good about the magnificent job being done. It's not magnificent, it's mediocre. One American doctor beating the bush to visit one sick Montagnard in his hut isn't so wonderful when you consider that the doctor hasn't supplies or adequate medications, lacks the authority to initiate reforms, and can't communicate this to the higher levels.

Visitors from Project Concern are here and Stan and I have been briefing them. I'm skeptical but will lay it on the line. The sanitary conditions are unchanged here after 6 months. People lie on the floor while we've a warehouse of empty beds. Despite how we look on paper we are impotent. We haven't authority. Our roles and status is as unstructured and ambiguous as when we arrived. The most unhappy part has been our inability to communicate this. People talk of their own training programs for Montagnards in elementary health and first aid. But without supplies they are useless in the hamlets. Then there's the problem of getting people to accept medicine and techniques. "Ah," says Project Concern. "No problem. We take Montagnards and place them in Montagnard villages with their own people." "Ah," says I. "Not so in Darlac province." I explained how, at Lac Thien, the rural health workers practiced in their home villages but still faced resistance! Of course in Project Concern Hospitals and training centers they don't share our problems. They pay their own staff. I explained that Dr. Niem has no control over the jobs of his staff who are on a government payroll. There is no supervisory structure. (I feel like the Ancient Mariner.)

Ban Me Thuot Headlines

An American whose enlistment and tour in Vietnam expired several weeks ago is being held over for investigation. He'd burned his ID card and renounced his U.S. citizenship up in Pleiku.

An American Air Force Sgt. is being sent back to the states. He couldn't handle his alcohol.

I sat down last week and wrote a critique about the MILPHAP mission. It was triggered by a booklet recently published by USAID describing all the projects going on here in Darlac province, very long and complete, even listing the interpreters hired by their office, two American girls who'd arrived 2 weeks ago from the International Volunteer Service to teach

Montagnards, but there was no mention of our work. (Since then USAID people have suffered guilt and apologized.)

Stan and I attended a sacrifice in our honor so I've a second Montagnard bracelet. Deep down I enjoy the hospitality of the Montagnard despite detesting their rice wine. They laugh, talk, touch you. It's dark and smoky inside the long house but you feel like its home. The Vietnamese officials I've met are quite the opposite. At their social gatherings you feel stiff and uncomfortable.

There was some action last night. Bill and I were lying in bed and talking about the Vietnam problem when we reached the question, is Communism a threat to me? At that instant mortars began falling to the west of us, about quarter mile away, and machine gun fire. We grabbed our clothes and gear and went to our stations. Then the siren. Blackness and running feet and weapons clicking. Afterwards, in our quarters again, we agreed that, at this time and at this place, Communism was a threat to us. What happened was the V.C. tried to mortar the airstrip of the Aviation Company. (Rounds fell short and onto the road and the plantation. Some hit the runway but nobody and no planes got hit. But mortars and small arms near the dam hurt people at Buon K'Ser. 8 killed, 17 wounded.)

The surgery ward has as many people on the floor as in beds (2–3 per bed). It's filthy and crowded as always. But carrying out reforms inhibits interpersonal relations. You can't have it both ways and the priority these days is making friends.

I didn't get to work on the casualties of last night. Too busy running the clinic and Stan's ward (he's on a mobile trip to Buon Blick) and the VD Program. Police round up the prostitutes and bring them to the hospital in a truck and I screen them for disease. On Stan's ward a 3 month-old baby was given Chinese medicine before coming to the hospital. She was half paralyzed when she got here; died within hours. A girl was admitted with typhoid fever and perforated bowel; she died the same day. I got my hands on some Chinese medicine back in Buon Anur (Buon Ho district) and will send it to Tokyo for analysis.

Stan just came back from a week at Buon Blick. It was his first mobile trip, 5 days. (Bill also took a 3-day trip to Buon Y Yang.) Stan was unshaven, filthy and wearing a camouflaged uniform with a parachute the Special Forces out there gave him. (I'd taken over his ward for the week and was impressed with how smoothly it ran.)

We've all gone on mobile trips now. Stan, our CO, really can't leave that much and Bill is our only surgeon. That limits their traveling. All the doctors in the province are in this city, 14 military and 3 American (not counting 2 American doctors attached to American units here, MACV and *the 155th Aviation Company). But the real need is in the districts. That's where they beg for counter-insurgency efforts. RVN doctors won't go out so that's what we're here for. So I go out.*

The Vietnamese charity ward has been razed and replaced with a totally different structure completed in 2 weeks time. Sheet metal roof, no windows, hot and dark. Not what we would have recommended.

My recommendations and criticisms about our mission continue to go into my reports. I really don't think anyone reads them.

There is an expression, to "piss into the wind," an image quite clear and vivid. The question for our mission was, given what we were learning, why did I persist at trying to alert my superiors? Why "piss into the wind"? Aside from the immediate relief, I don't know. There must be a pressure building up (to follow the pissing metaphor), enough to make finding relief a priority, even knowing I'll get all stinky right afterwards. Because I was, thus, "relieving myself," it probably didn't matter if anyone read my reports. Howling, like gratuitous violence, doesn't seem to be about communication. It seems to be more about expelling a toxin.

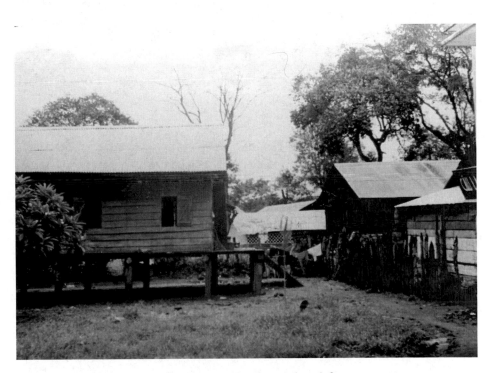

Old Vietnamese charity ward on left.

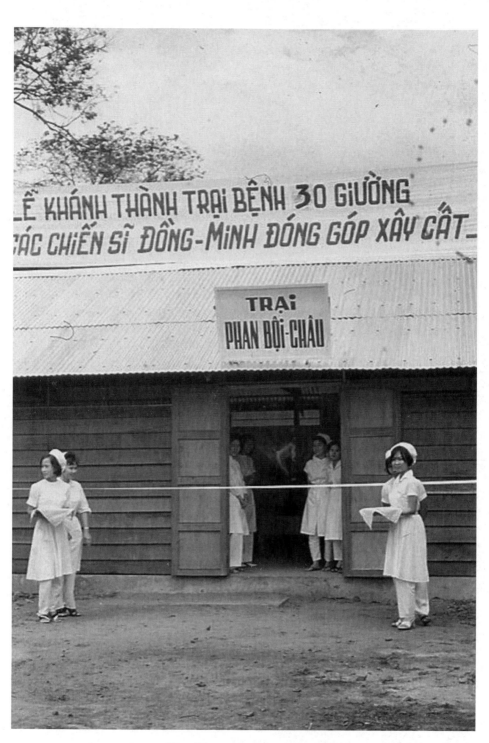

New Vietnamese charity ward.

Eyes on An Lac
(and the Ground, Too)

I flew to An Lac the other day for a look-see and talk with the Special Forces there who'll be my host for a several weeks mobile trip. On the way back we made some visual reconnaissance. Phantom jets were striking a V.C. village. We tuned into their radio frequency and followed the attack from our vantage point in the sky. Then we heard the Phantom jets radio for the VN Air Force to come in. Just about had to beg. VN Air Force had all kinds of excuses, but the visibility was excellent. They couldn't cop out. Then, over Lac Thien, we tuned into an ambush. We had flown over the pass earlier but had seen nothing. Two dead, 6 wounded, all strikers caught by two V.C. companies. We watched the chopper drop down to evacuate the wounded.

Two-Faced Soldier,
Back with a Vengeance

A private—the soldier I'd med evac'd to psychiatrists at Nha Trang not long ago [see chapter 7]—he'd since returned, "fit for duty" and is now assigned to the MACV radio shack at the Bungalow, was supposed to be on duty at midnight. He showed up drunk at the gate at 1:00 A.M. with a weapon, a clip in it, and a round in the chamber. Now, in our Bungalow compound, all weapons must be "cleared," that is, unloaded prior to entrance. He went to Detachment HQ. There the men on duty took the weapon from him and sent for the lieutenant colonel. When a courier entered the office and stood between the night orderly and the weapon, the private snatched it back, reloaded it, slipped it on automatic, and lined the men there against the wall. "I could kill you all," he said. Then he backed out the door whereupon the men on duty turned off the lights, locked the door, and ducked behind desks with their own weapons. Then the private returned. He banged and forced the door open, breaking the lock. The sergeant raised his rifle and fired point blank at the private but it misfired. The click of the trigger broke the silence and the private, thank God, didn't turn loose on them. He backed out again and went into the shadows across the courtyard. When he was captured and the situation under control the sergeant went upstairs to my room. He knew of my prior consultations with the private. The sergeant, a medic at the dispensary here, was shaking and white. I gave him a glass of ice-water. I was awake by now, listening.

I went downstairs. The colonel was there and the now disarmed private was really off. Because I've no authority over the American soldiers here I first asked the colonel if I could be of help. He said, no. The sergeant just groaned. MPs were called and they took the private to the Aviation Company for the night (we've no guardhouse). Today he's on his way back to the psychiatrist at the 8th Field Hospital in Nha Trang. (What will it take, manslaughter?)

Following this second (his third?) trip to Nha Trang and the 8th Field Hospital, the psychiatrists were still unimpressed. He was to return to BMT, medically cleared, which meant he was responsible for his actions and therefore would never make it to BMT. He was placed under arrest, and I was called to testify at his pre-court-martial hearing. At deposition they learned I had neither psychiatric credentials nor training and lost interest in me. I didn't have to leave my work to travel to testify at his court-martial. I was glad.

Harmony: Found and Lost

The province chief, his staff, and people from USAID, Sector (MACV), and MILPHAP, met for cocktails at the province chief's home. Later, high school girls (VN and Montagnard) came to the Bungalow along with VN dignitaries. Speeches, gifts, cards of greeting to all of us. The most beautiful part was a Christmas Pageant put on by the "Young Rhade People, Protestant Church of Ban Me Thuot." The missionaries arranged the show and it was first class. In a series of 9 brief scenes, with beautiful costumes these young people re-enacted the Christmas story, from the prophesy of Micah to Herod's anger and the family fleeing, all in the Rhade language.

Best of all were the songs between scenes sung in one, two, and three-part harmony, also in Rhade. Some were familiar carols and other were new and beautiful melodies. We never saw the last scene. The colonel, who'd left briefly, came in and announced: "Please, don't anyone panic. We have serious reason to believe the city is in danger tonight. All staff report to my office. All soldiers go immediately to your rooms and prepare for Alert. The civilians are welcome to spend the night here at the Bungalow. The Montagnards will be escorted home."

And so the show ended, without even a chance for applause. That night we slept in our clothes. Nothing happened. Intelligence had reported a V.C. regiment digging in outside town. But, by 7:00 A.M. the V.C. truce was in effect and things were back to normal.

At An Lac Special Forces "A" Camp
the Day After Christmas

I'm at An Lac at a Special Forces camp on a bluff overlooking a pretty river. On the map it's south of Ban Me Thuot where the three provinces, Darlac, Quang Duc, and Tuyen Duc, meet. The people in the villages around us are Montagnards, the Rhade, Mnung, and Koho (K'haw); the last live in circular houses on the ground, not long-houses on pillars like Rhade. Koho have no written language and are not as sophisticated as the Rhade. As yet, no plan of action. After a few days observing I'll outline a program and set to work. 8,000 tribesmen life here in scattered villages.

In his attempt to make up for neglecting us the USAID rep promised all sorts of cooperation beginning with a helicopter lift of my medical supplies and personal clothing to An Lac, supposedly last Saturday. So I deposited these items at the USAID office as requested and here I am with no sign of my supplies, the clothes on my back, toilet kit, and weapon. I've radioed back. [How easily I'd forget the exigencies of wartime. How quickly I'd forget how, each in his or her own way, was doing the best he or she could. But, doctor's are, almost by nature, problem-solvers, fixers, and reformists, our asset and our liability.]

The weather is good, the food excellent, the water drinkable, my quarters number one. The mail plane comes irregularly. Don't worry about me. We're miles from everywhere and things are quiet. The camp is a fortress.

I make my rounds among the hamlets and villages, covering them pretty thoroughly. I leave leeway for follow-up visits. The health of the tribesmen is better than I'd expected although there was an extraordinary amount of pig tape-worm. I'd instruct them to cook the pork longer. There's never been a doctor in this area so I may remain several weeks. I'd sometimes swim in the river before lunch time. I think the villagers at Buon Eatul are planning a party for me.

The Special Forces Camp (as well as the villages) lie along this river which flows northwest into Cambodia and, at places, one must cross by ferry, a small wooden craft connected to an elevated cable across the river. A ferryman poles the boat across. I also made trips by jeep to the hamlets with a truck of strikers for security.

Harmony: Found and Celebrated

I enjoy my work here. Mornings I work in the Special Forces built hospital—10 beds—located in the village down the hill. I am accompanied by the midwife, Co San, who serves as interpreter. She is a widow. Afternoons I take a medical patrol on hamlet rounds. The Montagnards, mixed Mnung and Koho, prefer colorful bracelets and beaded necklaces, earlobes are pierced and stretched to shoulder length, and many men tie their hair back in a bun. We travel by jeep, by river ferry, walk trails, and wade waist-deep across swift streams. There are enough supplies now.

Yesterday afternoon the Special Forces invited the village chiefs and dignitaries for an "American Style" nampay party. We made a mixture of apple cider, bourbon, gin, vodka, and champagne. This time we presented bracelets, shiny new ID bracelets with the names of the chief and his village engraved. Much singing, gong playing, laughing. The guest list was interesting. Tribesmen missing ears, fingers, teeth, and wearing old French War hats, bandanas, V.C. shirts. Three of the guests were Vietcong captured several months ago. They're now our allies. After they were captured the Special Forces brought them to camp and treated them to their first bread, butter, and meat in many years.

During the festivities the captain of the VN Special Forces team here (called LLDB and that works in combination with the American SF Team), himself Rhade, tried to do the twist. The Sgt. went among the Montagnards with his tape recorder recording songs, impromptu speeches, toasts — everyone having a terrific time. A helicopter came in unexpectedly and two visiting Special Forces majors and their party looked around, quite nervous and nonplused. They left pretty quick. I wonder what their impressions were. (They came from the SP "C" Team on the coast, quite out of touch with the "A" teams who go native at the drop of a hat.)

Late at night when everyone left, some SF people, myself, Koho interpreters and a VN midwife and cook sat in the mess-hall drinking scotch. I found a guitar and we Americans began singing. We harmonized to, "Try to Remember," "The Cruel War," and "When Johnny comes Marching Home." Then the girls sang VN songs, war songs about the girl who laments she is not with her lover-soldier and asks who will carve her name on his rifle stock, who will cut lilies for her from the jungle trail. It's been a long time since I've sung. We sit on the border of Darlac and Tuyen Duc Province with no roads in or out. We're not even on the map.

Christmas Truce 1966

Christmas Day was a day of truce. I went with a small armed convoy to the distant village of Dam Ron, a trip that took almost an hour. Along

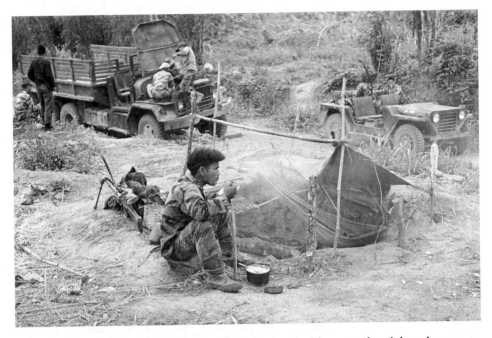

Our convoy pauses at a counter-ambush site that had been set the night prior to our trip deeper into the district.

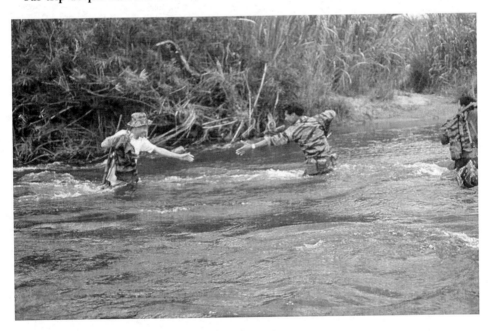

En route to Dakao.

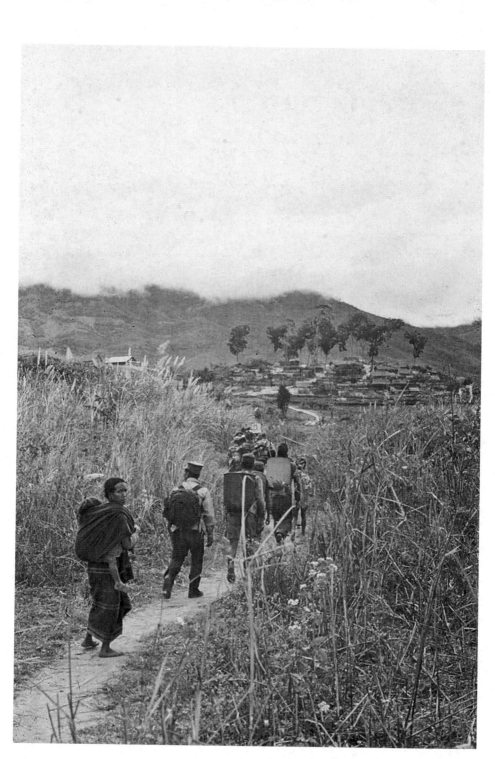

The hamlet of Dakao.

the way we passed the sites of old ambushes. We found trenches the V.C. had built for future ambushes. I went along to hold sick call. Because one truck was having engine difficulties and kept lagging behind we stopped. There was, off the track, a striker casually eating. He was one of 6 who'd been sent out the day before to set up a counter-ambush position and guard the road. Ahead was a bridge and these security guards were there to keep the V.C. away from the bridge.

The truck started up and we continued but, once again, it pooped out. No one was happy about being stuck like this in this place. The truck finally started up again and turned back, dropping men off along the way. (When we eventually return to base we picked up those men who watched for V.C.)

The last leg of the trip was on foot with 2 streams to ford carrying our supplies on poles between us. A very strong current pulled one of the men off and under the water but he pulled himself out further downstream. So, with wet clothing and soggy boots we all finally came in sight of Dakao, a hamlet situated on a hill top in the distance like some fairy-tale city. (Because the sub-district HQ is in the larger village of Dam Ron nearby we referred to this trip as the "Dam Ron" trip.)

Preparing for sick call the patients lined up outside the aid station to see me and it was during this sick call I discovered an elderly Koho man dying. So, on the Jan 1 truce we made a return trip and carried the old man back to An Lac and flew him to Ban Me Thuot. I returned to BMT soon afterwards and continued to take care of him. He was dying of metastatic cancer. It was important that he be home when he passed so I went begging for a chopper. A Vietnamese Air Force plane took him home.

Monkey Business and Perimeter Checks

I enjoyed playing with a monkey. He'd sit in my arms and spend hours pulling the hair on my arms. I think it was an instinct because amongst themselves they pick lice from one another's hair. Once in a while he'd yank hard and I'd say "Ouch!" and his eyebrows would jump and he'd murmur "Hmmmm?" He'd look terribly concerned and shift his body a bit, all without interrupting his hair pulling.

The Special Forces are short-handed now. I'm to take my shift at night guard duty. It means periodic communications check with the "B" Team at BMT, making sure the short-wave radio is working, walk the perimeter and check the guards. Are they awake? Are their weapons loaded? I explained that I never had radio training and know little about weapons. They said that was OK. So, just like being on duty as an intern, you hope you don't get called. I'll make my rounds with a VN Special Forces soldier because, god-forbid when we're challenged by the perimeter guards I might have forgotten the counter-sign to their pass-word challenge. (They are all Rhade numbers.)

I'd like to remain here the rest of the month but they'll no longer need me after this week. With that in mind I've been preparing for the next trip, either Ban Don, a Special Forces camp far to the northwest of Ban Me Thuot near the Cambodian border, or back to Lac Thien. Now we wait for a med evac helicopter to take a patient out. It took some doing just to get the patient into the camp. We took him from his village 30 kilometers away and marched with the litter though jungle and across deep streams. The final leg of the journey was the flight to Dalat. We've been 3 days waiting for that plane. If he dies after coming this far without reaching a hospital I'm sure the Montagnards will never again allow us to evacuate one of their own.

Whenever a chopper comes in I'll go home. During these past weeks I held sick call mornings in the makeshift dispensary the Special Forces built long ago. Afternoons I took a medical patrol on village rounds. I came here alone and had plenty of help from Vietnamese medics and Koho medics-in-training. That way I was able to do a little teaching. I tell the tribespeople that their VN government sent me here to help them. (That's pretty close to the truth.) Actually, their government has no health personnel out here and the entire medical program is in the hands of our Special Forces and they pay the medics plus the midwife, plus use their American supply channels. There are plenty of medicines and the people work hard, unlike BMT where many nurses are government appointed, no one can fire them, they work at their own pace, and they don't take instruction. Here I'm forever explaining, teaching.

Security is from the strikers, Koho and Mnung tribesmen, some as young as 12 years old. The commanding officer, a captain of the Vietnamese Special Forces Team is Rhade. Much of the camp is underground; bunkers, trenches, and tunnels. And, like all such "A" Camps, there is an escape route. In the event the V.C. attack the village of the dependents (the location of the dispensary) and, using villagers as hostages, approach and demand the Americans (and this has happened at other places), the 7 Americans must slip out. A trench leads to a passage under the barbed wire and to the river. There are several boats and a current should carry them to Lac Thien.

I visited a Koho hamlet, Rochae, and another, Romin. We needed a ferry service.

It's cold at night. We've had lots of rain and the river is swollen and fast. Here in the mountains it feels cold like Maine in November.

My trip home from An Lac was by helicopter at treetop level all the way. As always I'm both winded and full of pep.

10

Fault Lines:
Honor, Trust and Caring

A "Hush-Hush" Story

There is an article in the November Saturday Evening Post about a Special Forces "A" Camp. (The guys here enjoyed it.) The article mentioned that Green Berets are sitting on the hottest story over here, civil war. I'm surprised they wrote about it; it's confidential, about the tension between Montagnard and Vietnamese. Suffice to say that the patrol that just returned here after 17 days out had a hairy story to tell. They were fired upon by South Vietnamese forces at Dalat and it wasn't mistaken identity either! It was deliberate! But that's another story and better kept hush-hush for the time being. One gets to see and hear much which never reaches outside ears. Please don't mention this incident.

More Ban Me Thuot Headlines

We've a new doctor here, a Project VIETNAM physician. He left his practice to volunteer 2 months here, Doctor Hugh Auchincloss, professor of surgery at Columbia P&S, a gentle, generous, and sincere man. (His wife is sister of McGeorge Bundy and he's a cousin to Jacqueline Kennedy, related to her by marriage. Jackie's mother married an Auchincloss.)

Today Dr. Grimsley arrived to work at the hospital. He's a civilian physician from North Carolina; has been here several years under USAID auspices. Didn't like his desk job. Fought to get reassigned here.

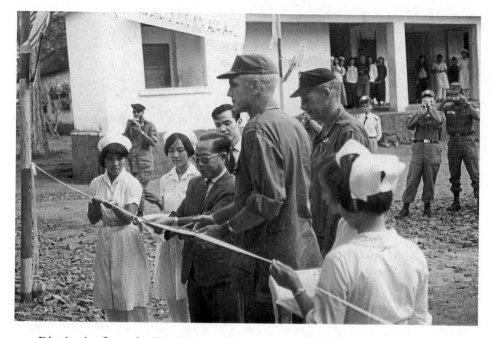

Dignitaries from the Dar Lac province government, "Sector" (MACV), and the Ban Me Thuot hospital attended the ribbon cutting for the new charity ward. Rhade nurse H Nhe is on the far left; Lt. Henry Brown is behind her in background; Dr. Niem is fifth figure from left; and Col. David Silver, MACV Senior Advisor, is sixth from left.

At a Conference in Nha Trang with medical representatives from all over the country it was announced that, of the 23 MILPHAP teams working in-country, ours is one of the three said to be successful. Has someone been putting in a good word for us? Has publicity of the success of the new charity ward reached the conferees in Nha Trang? (A doctor from one of the Air Force MILPHAP teams is a patient at the psychiatric hospital there.)

Albert Einstein Alumni have sent a total of 15 boxes of supplies all received. With these new supplies maybe I can realize my ambition to make my mobile trips mixed American-Vietnamese teams.

I ran into Special Forces Captain Jackson (from Lac Thien) this morning. He's in Ban Me Thuot; leaves for home tomorrow to get married and, perhaps, leave the army. A good man.

It's now very, very cold [January 1967], something they neglected to mention at Fort Sam Houston. Not much sun, either.

There are improvements in the wards at the hospital in Ban Me Thuot and supplies much more realistic. Five months to go.

In March our first MILPHAP replacement doctor arrives and those 3

American nurses. My opinion? Too many cooks. The problem is getting some of the Vietnamese nurses to do their work. The VN Army doctors complained about us and asked that we leave Seems we were cutting into their private practices in town. The point is, if those 14 doctors assumed responsibility for the civilian hospital and provided coverage for the districts we would leave.

April I'll go to Hong Kong for R&R.

Rest easy. I was nowhere near the Iron Triangle. You were looking at An Loc. I was at An Lac, further to the north. It's near Phi Di Ya and inside Darlac Province.

Work in the Ban Me Thuot outpatient clinic is so different. The two male VN technicians there now are eager to learn and I'm having a good time.

Dr. Lou Fishman, Air Force (NY) flew in for a day. (I'd met him at Lac Thien.) He lives on the seashore in a French villa yet envies me because all he treats are U.S. Airmen for colds and sore backs. He suggested I fly to Nha Trang for sun and swimming. It sounds good. TET (February 8) is next week and a truce and I'll be going to Ban Don.

Presenting symptoms of intestinal parasites can be: eating dirt, urge to drink gasoline, bad dreams, dysaesthesia of certain body surfaces.

The V.C. ambushed some civilians on the road to Buon Ho. Pretty bad.

I'm proud of what I'm doing here. When I come home that feeling comes with me. Not really surprised that time passes quickly. I no longer try to change the scene. But, somehow, things have happened, like a new ward, new constructions, other renovations underway. Medicine donations from home help so much, like with hemorrhoids, sinusitis, moniliasis, heart failure, and so-called "incurable" skin diseases.

Mobile Trip to Quang Nhieu (Where Vietcong Provide Security?)

I returned this morning from a week in Quang Nhieu, about 25 km. north of Ban Me Thuot. There are no Americans stationed there so we lived in a small, triangular Regional-Popular Forces compound, total strength 1 company. Ate C rations and bathed in a stream, and shaved with the jeep's mirror, shivering and chattering. I took along Hoan and one man, Pfc. Aragon. The health of the people there is pretty poor and the only reason I didn't stay longer was security.

I'm busy, eating well—the long-johns keep me warm at night as I have only one blanket. I take my turn on night guard duty checking outposts calling Ban Me Thuot to make sure the radios are OK, but without the blundering I'd written about from An Lac. I live in a tent.

I lived in a med dugout and it was the roughest trip I'd taken. I'm still constipated. The "hole in the ground" we used was outside the fort and beyond the moat that surrounds the fort. At the edge of the tall grass there mixed with barbed wire and mines was the "hole" in an area about 10 feet wide. It was the most insecure camp I've seen. The enemy can get within throwing range of the compound and still be outside the wires plus out of sight. So, between the rustling grass on the one side and the machine gun ports facing me across the moat— and this is what really tightened the sphincters and kept me constipated— the various patrols and outposts communicating with one another by rifle shot kept me from relaxing enough to move my bowels. One try was enough. I put my heart into it but, when those shots came I just pulled up drawers and hurried back and never went again.

At the dispensary in town I kept my weapon on the table with the medicines. The Popular Forces stationed guards all around but, out at Quan Nhieu, many of these Popular Forces are V.C.

I took precautions on the road back to Ban Me Thuot. A squad of soldiers preceded us in a truck and we drove in their dust cloud as fast as we could in our open jeep. To be less conspicuous as an American I wore my black pajamas on the trip and sandals and a bullet-proof vest. Anyone looking to sight an American would have had to get up pretty close; we were all brown with dust.

That mobile trip to Quang Nhieu was a last-minute inspiration of the province chief's. There was a big operation in progress in the north and refugees were moving towards Quang Nhieu and the province chief asked for a medical team. At first a 4-man Vietnamese team went but the province chief pulled them after one day. (He prefers medics around him to impress people and he was going to Dat Le so he took them to Dat Le.) My trip was a propaganda show. What disease can you cure in one visit? So everyone gets shots but no one gets cured. Unfortunately, if anything, you just build up a person's resistance to whatever drug you inject. I was asked to follow-up. On one day's notice we loaded the jeep and raced out. It was poorly planned, of course, but, nonetheless, a successful trip. I was glad we made the return trip. But Quang Nhieu is crawling with V.C. The Mewal Plantation (French, coffee) is a nest for them. And the jeep run through the plantation always gave me sweaty palms. I don't want to go through that any more. I'm scared. Maybe two more mobile trips.

Next week I leave for a Special Forces Camp at Ban Don for several weeks. Interesting. In the beginning I couldn't get volunteers for my mobile trips. I had to pick my men. Now I'm over-subscribed. Too many have asked to go along. I must say no. The men are eager to go into the districts. But it's getting near the end and now I'm getting cold feet. I'll take 2 medics and stay 2–4 weeks. Yes, these mobile trips are vogue.

Tet in Ban Me Thuot, 1967

I pitched a 22–3 victory in softball and hit the ball a lot and got sun-burned. My nose is pretty raw. I got feeling a little lightheaded and nauseated so I drank saltwater. Could be I got salt-depleted from all the running around in the sun.

It's getting warmer [February 9, 1967] I'm tanned from playing vol-leyball at siesta time (noon to 3:00 p.m.). It's TET and we've the next 3 days off. It's the beginning of the lunar year and spring. The team gave out cards and gifts and many of us have been invited to the homes of VN friends. The nights have been noisy with firecrackers and weapons firing into the air. During the day the marketplace is deserted; many people out walking with families, dressed in newest and best clothing. I was especially pleased to receive a card from Y Rulick, medical chief of the Lac Thien dispensary.

First World Meets Third World: More American Gaffes

We, the MILPHAP doctors, were invited to a luncheon in our honor by Montagnard dignitaries. The day of the luncheon we deliberately avoided lunch in the Bungalow mess. One didn't want to give offense by refusing food because of lack of appetite. We were directed to take seats at the end of a small, open, conference-like room while, before us, a half-dozen or more Montagnard men squatted. Plates with cut up chicken were given to us. Words were spoken (we came with no translator) and gestures indicated we begin. We smiled and, slowly, with our fingers, began eating. But something was wrong. It didn't feel right. And as we'd eat the men before us began inching forward, towards us, not taking eyes off us. Banach caught on and held out his plate and gestured that they come forward and share. The effect was instantaneous — electric — as if the ice was broken, as if a circle had been completed. They approached and we shared. We'd been so off target; it was so embarrassing. We did not know that the Montagard diet customarily is low in meat. (I never spoke about it let alone wrote about it until now.)

Pfc. Melberg tells this story (from the Lac Thien mobile trip):

"I seem to remember an incident when we were being welcomed to a vil-lage with rice wine. It was in one of the long thatched houses on stilts with cut-out windows at floor level. We took turns drinking rice wine from a jug in the center of the room through a long reed. As we would drink, a man sitting on the other side of the jug would refill it with water from a tin can. I think it was to keep track of how much we drank. Since we, as guests, drank first, our wine was the most potent. After my turn I went back to take my place along the wall. I was a little off. When I leaned back I went right out the window. I remember lying on my back looking up at a water buffalo that was under the house for shade [Daniel Melberg, personal communication].

When an Opposite Number Doesn't Compute

A Mnung tribesman was flown in from Quang Duc province with his sick daughter. She was admitted to the Montagnard charity ward (covered by the VN civilian woman doctor). Stan accidentally worked up the kid but properly turned the case over to the civilian doctor when he discovered his error. He said he'd pay the bill if the kid stayed on his own ward. "No." Stan said he had all the necessary medications. "No." He offered the doctor the medicine. "No." Today some pilots told me that a Montagnard and child had been living in the empty hangar for the past 4 days. The kid looked pretty sick. I drove out and got the story. After 9 days in the hospital the doctor, my Vietnamese counterpart, told the man he'd have to buy his medicines in town. (This medicine, incidentally, is available in the hospital pharmacy. But it's long been the custom for nurses and VN doctors to say, "fini," when their ward is out. They don't go the pharmacy for refills and the pharmacy doesn't check.) Many times Stan finds a patient hasn't been receiving medication — "We're out," says the nurse. "But it's in the pharmacy," Stan points out. The nurse denies this. Stan goes to the pharmacy and brings back the medicine. "See," he tells her, "we've plenty." No comment. (This agony has been standard operating procedure since last July.) Anyhow, even if the hospital were out we have plenty of substitutions in the samples sent us still not used. But my doctor-counterpart doesn't communicate with us. So this Montagnard, in loin cloth and with hair back in a bun ... he didn't have any money ... so his doctor sent him packing.

I drive my jeep to the airstrip on the outskirts of town. There, in the hangar, are the tribesman and his sick daughter, just as the pilot said. I confirm she is the patient who'd been discharged four days ago from the hospital Montagnard charity ward due to continued lack of medicines (and they had no money to buy the medicine in town as directed). The child's condition, deteriorating from lack of adequate food and water, from malnutrition, dehydration, and starvation, is now certain to deteriorate further because, unknown to her father, planes from the 155th no longer fly to Quang Duc from whence they'd come several weeks earlier. I drive the girl and her father back to the hospital and place her in the pay ward this time, as some GIs have offered to pay for her care. The medicines she needs are available at the pay ward and in stock in the hospital pharmacy.

When an Opposite Number Doesn't Compute II

One of the casualties of the ambush on the road to Buon Ho was a priest. He was shot. The VN Army surgeon operated. The man suddenly went into shock, no blood pressure, no pulse. Dr. Auchincloss happened by, saw the patient on the operating table and no one else in sight. He dashed to the refrigerator and got blood and began running it into the patient. During the second pint the Vietnamese surgeon returned. After first ripping the intravenous blood tube out of the man's arm he blew his stack. Yes, he knew the man was in shock. He stormed out. Dr. Auchincloss got another unit of blood and started it running.

The man's alive and recuperating on Stan's ward. His blood pressure and pulse are stable. Dr. Auchincloss is still shaken by this incident. [P. A New York Times *article, January 25, 1967, p. 2, written by a Mr. Apple who was in Ban Mc Thuot, had featured Dr. Auchincloss.] But it came as no surprise to us. In my view, when the VN doctors say the patient comes first it's lip service. I note that, as there are now more modern supplies, more drugs and affluence in the civilian hospital, the price for staying on the pay-ward has doubled. Also, as things have improved, a "service" charge is attached to out-patients who have X-Rays taken, even though the X-Ray film is supplied free by the U.S. Charity patients are still sent packing if they can't afford to buy drugs in town even as the drugs are in the hospital pharmacy. (The hospital says it's out of them.) The ward doctor won't ask for more and the pharmacist won't volunteer there are more. As a result, mountains of the stuff sit gathering dust in the pharmacy while nurses on the ward smile and say "fini" and send patients to buy the same stuff in town.*

American taxpayers pay so the VN peasant will have medical care and all this makes it difficult. Streptomycin lines the pharmacy shelves while plague patients die a lingering death on the ward because a nurse doesn't go and get more when she runs out. (The MILPHAP have no say in administration, programs, or reforms. This was built into the program design.) Authorities in Nha Trang and Saigon don't get the picture because they send directives to initiate this or that program. Our zeal to help was blunted long ago. If it wasn't we'd have stepped on far more toes and been totally black-balled. We swallow our anger (and our Hippocratic Oath). I hope tonight's movie is a comedy.

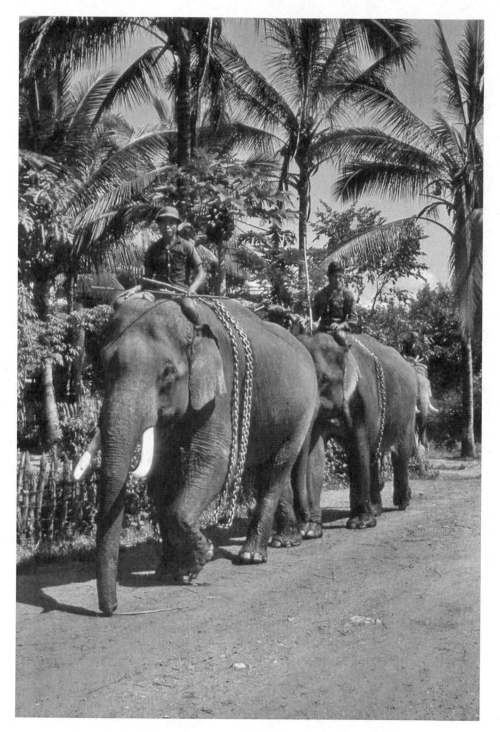

Working elephants with their Montagnard handlers.

Mobile Trip to Ban Don

I brought along Pfc. Aragon with me—he was with me at Quang Nhieu in January 1967 at that village 25 km north of Ban Me Thuot. He'd volunteered for this one. Also Sgt. Strickland, the most qualified medic on our team. He didn't want to come, threatened transferring out of MILPHAP if he was made to come. (Had this handsome and affable soldier gone off and found a mistress in town?) There are elephants out here, and peacocks, bear, leopards and tigers. The people are Mnung and Koho, also some Cambodian and Thai tribesmen.

Ban Don is west of BMT, about 20 miles from Cambodia. It's moderately hilly with scrub brush, trees, wood—not real jungle. Plenty of flat ground and rivers. Reminds me of pictures of Africa. Dirt roads, very dusty. Days are very hot and nights terribly cold. It consists of 2 villages, one Mnung, the other Laotian Montagnard, sitting on a river. There are several hamlets up to 10 km. in one direction. There is a government dispensary in town manned by one man, a Laotian Montagnard. He works for the South VN government, for Dr. Niem. I went to Ban Don with my 2 MILPHAP medics to help him out.

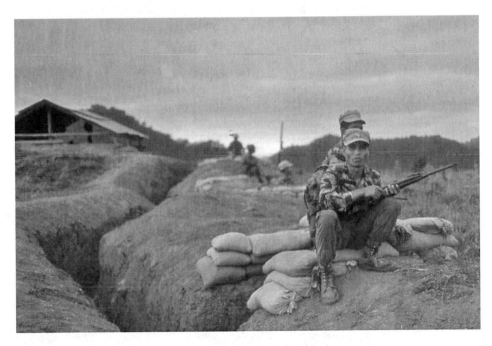

A weapons check before dark.

The Special Forces provide good security. Their camp isn't completed so the Special Forces team and the 3 companies of Montagnard strikers live alongside the air strip in tents. The new camp, still being built, is a mile away, very impressive with high, earthwork defenses. This place where I am had no perimeter except dirt mounds with strikers standing watch. Checking these defense positions at night, walking around with a flashlight, feels like being a duck at the shooting-gallery. I am very uneasy.

Planes come and go and great dust clouds settle on the camp. You walk and kick up dust 3 feet in the air. Jeeps and animals. Your eyes smart and you cough. At night it was the coldest I've experienced in-country. I'm quite tan and suffer a head cold.

Things went OK at first. The Special Forces-trained (Montagnard) medics helped me. We held sick call in the dispensary, a tiny, one-room infirmary, in Ban Don. Then we'd cross the bridge into Buon Tre to make house-calls.

Food was shitty; the Special Forces ate off the land. Water was from the river with lots of chlorine added and it tasted like swimming pool water. There wasn't that much work for my MILPHAP medics so I let them go home to Ban Me Thuot after 5 days. But, as the strikers drank the water, so did I. Within days of arriving I was prostrate with diarrhea.

Rumors are in the air about peace. Also, watch for more trouble with Montagnards. FULRO feels they've been screwed. The pact they'd signed with Premier Ky hasn't produced any results. They were promised a Montagnard province chief for Darlac. They still have a Vietnamese province chief.

Follow-up: FULRO finally quit their war in 1992 when they turned themselves over to a U.N. peace-keeping force in Cambodia in the fall of that year. Of all the armed groups to fight the Communist Vietnamese, North and South, they'd apparently held out the longest.

Doctor Down

At the beginning of the 2nd week it suddenly became intolerably hot. I worked in the sun seeing patients at a hamlet one day and became heat exhausted. Then came symptoms of gastroenteritis. It was a horrible sensation of impending nausea and diarrhea with myalgias. Felt completely washed-out. I never actually vomited but had watery stools constantly; couldn't even look at food. I was pale and dizzy and terribly weak.

For the next few days I'd make it to sick call in the dispensary, sitting down while I worked. Then to the camp at noon. No food, again. Lie in my bunk, in that hot tent which retained all the heat, too weak to lift an arm. But I must lower the mosquito net before nightfall, I'd think. The effort felt too much. I hadn't the strength. Oh, God! I'll do it at 2:00 in the afternoon, I'd tell myself. Close my eyes. open them. It's 2:00 in the afternoon. I'll lower the net at 5:00, I'd promise and close my eyes. Open them, it's 5:00. I could have cried. Why wouldn't someone lower the net for me? And then, at 9:00 p.m., dark already, stomach gurgling, I'd force myself to sit up and pull that net down, sweating, and collapse back onto the bed. Then sun up. No breakfast but I had to go to work. For three days it was that awful. I'd lost weight. My ribs showed, my face was drawn.

House-Call on Elephant Back

I had told the Special Forces Team that I wanted to cover all the hamlets. The one which looked impossible was Buon Drang Phok, further west, about 10 km. from Cambodia. It's inaccessible except by foot trail. The Special Forces Team was taking a load of supplies, food, soap, gifts including blankets and toys, and my medical equipment. They were traveling by elephant so they got an extra one for me.

Two elephants were nursing mothers so their calves came along. Of course the Special Forces had to pay for them along with the adult elephants carrying the burdens. The animals were hired like you'd hire a horse and buggy. This was Thursday and I awoke feeling better. I even ate a bowl of cereal and drank a cup of coffee for breakfast, my first food in 3 days. I told them I was up to it. We loaded up. I had to climb from the hood of a 2.5 ton truck onto the elephant's head, then step over the elephant-handler and find a position among the supplies in the basket on the elephant's back. (Unlike Indian elephants, these Asian elephants do not kneel to enable a rider to mount.) I was interested to learn that the Special Forces had only recently, in the 1960s, begun using them, hiring them out from local Montagnards. I removed the shiny bars and insignias from my uniform that identified me as an officer, a captain, a doctor.

There was Special Forces Captain Jerry Walters, a State Department civilian who worked for Civic Affairs, a Mr. Reed (I think), my Montagnard medic, myself, and one British correspondent [Richard West]and one photographer [Phillips Jones-Griffiths]. Before setting out I made sure to stuff my fatigue pockets with salt tablets and anti-diarrhea pills plus a roll of toilet paper. Our departure was temporarily delayed when, suddenly, 8 helicopters flew into Ban Don to lift out a company of strikers. What was hap-

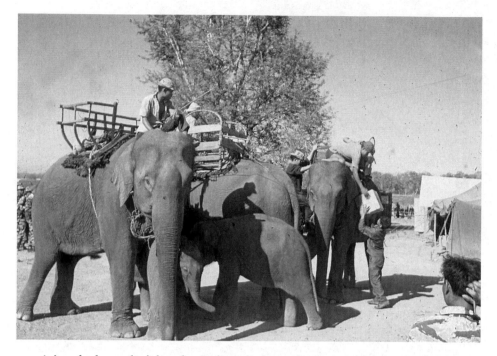

Asian elephants don't kneel as Indian elephants do. One mounted or loaded from the hood of a truck or from the ground. These elephants ran wild in the Central Highlands for centuries, and Montagnards had long been adept at catching and taming them. The property of the women, they were trained for transport of heavy items.

pening? Rumors said Buon Ho was being overrun by North Vietnamese regulars.

It was with this terrible news we set out. I was on the 3rd of 4 elephants. Behind me on the 4th elephant was a medic and a striker. I remember asking one of the correspondents when they'd arrived at camp, where in England he was from. "Actually, I'm from Wales." You could almost taste his accent.

It was 4 hours on the trail and the sun was incredibly hot. The calves kept close to their mothers as they were still nursing. Probably wouldn't be ready for work training for 2 or 3 years.

It was a long, long journey, crossing rivers, plodding forward alongside mountains. We reached tall cane and bamboo thickets after 3 hours when suddenly there was smoke and crackling sounds. A fire, a big one. The elephants got frightened. My driver went off the trail and we were really moving. Bamboo and cane were smacking my head and I couldn't see because I was forced to keep my head down with my arms covering my face. Every time we tried to return to the trail there was flames and crackling. Then

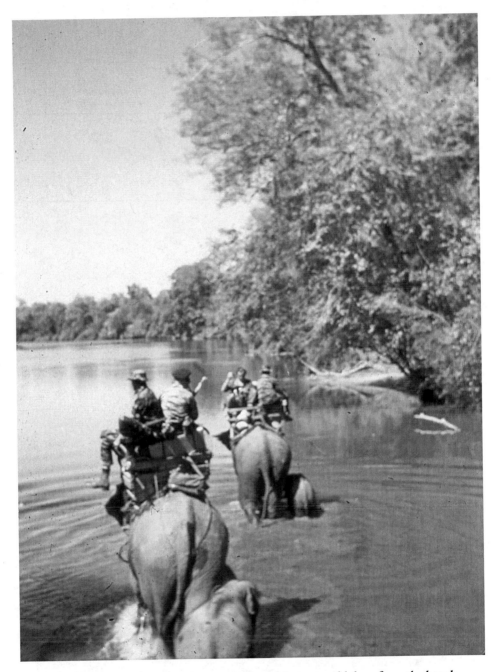

Serious discomfort for riders occurred when red ants would drop from the brush, after mild disturbance by the elephant's swaying motion, onto one's neck and shoulders.

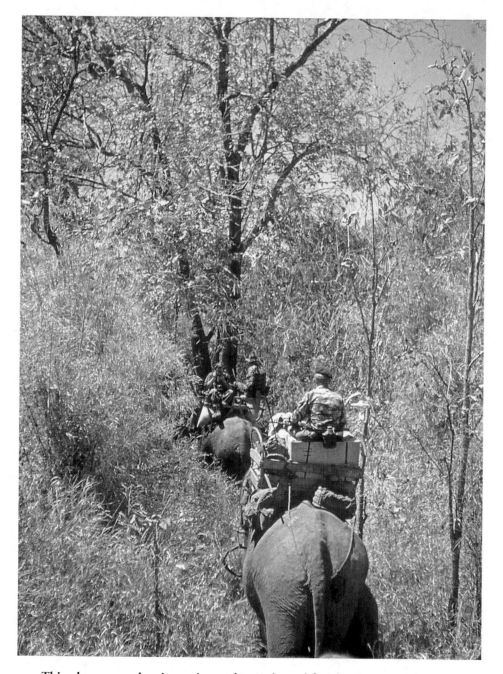

This photo was taken just prior to the smoke and fire that panicked the animals and sent them running in different directions. The fire, set by friends the day before to deter ambush, was evidently still smoldering on our approach.

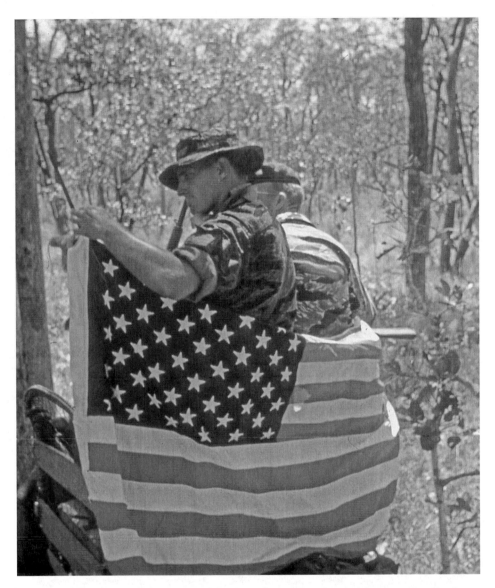

Because the Vietcong, having no helicopters, used elephants for conveying food and ammunition, it was common practice for suspecting American helicopter crews to fire on them. Our party's civic affairs civilian is securing the flag to protect us from friendly fire. (To his right is Special Forces Capt. Jerry Walters.)

we were in tall elephant grass. Finally, all the smoke was behind us. But there was no sign of the other animals, neither the ones ahead nor the one behind. We — the driver and me — were alone. For a second I had that fear that it had all been planned to separate me out from the others, and now I was lost. I knew compass direction and I'd checked a map before leaving and have worn a compass with my dog tags since arriving in Vietnam. I thought I could get back to Ban Don by myself.

After a long time and a lot of hollering, all the animals linked up. We got into Ban Drang Phok. My stomach was O.K. My mouth was dry. The water in my canteen was like swimming pool water. It burned. At the village I met the chief, shook hands all around. Before leaving I staggered to the river. The elephants were already there, bathing. Some women were washing. I just went down stream and took off all my clothes and fell in and it was heaven. That river was lifesaving.

The supplies were distributed and I'd held sick call and we headed home to Ban Don. To identify us as American, should we be spotted from the air and considered a V.C. convoy moving supplies and attacked, a U.S. flag was draped over one elephant's rump. It was 4:30 P.M. and we had to make camp before nightfall. The ride back, after 8 hours on elephant back (and this time my elephant was the lead elephant), you begin to hurt. I must have banged my L knee during the run through the cane breaks dodging the fire because it began throbbing when we got home after dark. My knee was swollen, red, and tender under the knee cap. [It remains tender to this day. Examinations have been negative. It's considered chronic tendonitis. I'd never connected it to that elephant ride until now, re-reading my letters.]

I held sick call today (Ban Don). Then took the first plane back to BMT. I don't want to go out anymore.

This story is iconic. I started off on a journey in considerable discomfort (the diarrhea with dehydration). The journey had unforeseen bumps and curves (the fire, smoke, and detour). It put me in harm's way (obliging a U.S. flag to be draped over the elephant's back to warn off American war planes). My presence did not have the intended effect (to inspire trust and enhanced allegiance to the government in power). Is this not America's story?

(My personal account, "Doctor to the Montagnards," was published in *Vietnam Magazine*, December 1999. An earlier account of it by Richard West had appeared in the *New York Times Magazine*, June 11, 1967, and conspicuously missing was any mention of the counter-ambush measure that backfired.)

Home to Ban Me Thuot and Sad News from Buon Ho: Reflections and Recovery

I came home from Ban Don, weak, underweight, and limping. Ban Me Thuot is strange; helicopters coming and going constantly. The Bungalow mess hall is deserted during meals.

The camp at Buon Ho held in the face of many North Vietnamese Army regulars, not V.C. Right now the enemy is bottled up and BMT and Special Forces, and Sector [the troops the MACV advised], and the RVN Division are involved. Even the L-19 planes used for visual reconnaissance are making rocket runs.

Instead of melting back into the jungle like the V.C. the NVN soldiers stood their ground and fought. They were wiped out. There were jet strikes and napalm. 42 enemy dead by body count. But my friend, Spec. 5 Powers, the medic at Buon Ho, was killed by machine-gun fire.

The V.C., to my knowledge, never bothered medics. I was never threatened, except for the vague bounty on the heads of MILPHAP doctors. We were already treating the guerrillas and their dependents as it was. But these North VN soldiers don't fool around. They are hard-core. But why in Darlac? Why now?

My visiting these villages and hamlets — usually the first doctor ever to visit them — means nothing if no one cares and the people are, after I leave, once again, dismissed, written off.

My strength is back, my appetite tripled, my spirits returned. My legs are OK and my vision cleared after stopping dysentery meds. But yesterday I had a typhoid inoculation which, with wine, leaves me feeling like I have dengue without the fever. I slept all day, achy and, again, weak and nauseated. I'm being recommended for the Bronze Star.

11

Fault Lines:
Health, Truth and Integrity

I Am Hospitalized

My symptoms returned — diarrhea, vomiting, gas, cramps, weight loss — and I was evacuated to the Eighth Field Hospital in Nha Trang. After observation for several weeks during which time the dysentery symptoms cleared, I asked to be discharged. No infectious agent was ever recovered from my stools despite repeated lab tests. My doctor there, Doctor Jose Segarra, had taken Basic with me and we had worked for a while together at the clinic at Wm. Beaumont Hospital in El Paso. We had both been assigned to MILPHAP and he had arrived in-country one month ahead of me. Unfortunately, at his assignment in a province in III Corps on the Cambodian border, he had come to lose considerable weight within 5 months and so had to quit the program. So we meet again, this time with me as his patient. Tests for worms, amebiasis, malaria, etc. were negative. My EKG was normal. Yet my weight was down from 185 lb. to 165 lb., a 20 lb. loss.

> What foresight my mother had to insist we children learn to type. Wherever I go there is a typewriter.
> I wear a blue hospital uniform. The ward is air-conditioned. There is fluorescent lighting, good food, nurses. My weight bounces around 170 lbs, sometimes higher, sometimes down, depending on the dysentery and how many times I'd barfed. Labs are abnormal with only hints at an etiology.
> The Red Cross takes patients to the beach afternoons so I get sunshine and I swim. Nha Trang has one of the most beautiful natural beaches I've

ever seen, big waves, pleasantly cool water, a VN canteen that sells beer and cokes. There are lifeguard towers. I'm very tan, very skinny, and have a Yul Brynner haircut. I enjoy this rest and the freedom from worries. There are no security problems. I'm relaxed and enjoy peace of mind. I haven't smoked for 8 days.

My work is farthest from my mind. Even the construction of the dispensary at Ban Don; I wanted to be in on that. I've my own ideas about design; I wanted to be part of the discussion. But it doesn't bother me.

Everyone here is American. No one has heard of Ban Me Thuot or Dar Lac Sector. It's difficult to explain what I do. The past 2 years build-up has been primarily of all–American units.

Sometimes I get the Asian edition of The Times and Newsweek so I know about RFK and his 6,000 word tone-poem about ending the bombing and the White House watchers stepping all over each other to see LBJ wince or fart or whatever he does. And LBJ follows through with some non-escalation escalation, like mining rivers and harbors and naval bombardments inside NVN territorial waters. What's it to be, RFK or LBJ? Stop the bombing and wait for a sign from Hanoi? Or lay it on hard?

During the great televised "teach-in" some time ago a psychiatrist was called upon by an investigating committee to give his views on this matter. He said that you don't change a man's beliefs by punishing him. On the contrary, his fervor, his zeal for his cause, is strengthened under duress. When I listened to this I agreed. But now I think differently. The purpose of the bombing isn't to force the enemy to abandon his ideology, just his proselytizing. Please, no bombing pauses until after I leave this country.

I read Letters to Editor, and supporters of LBJ speak out for "getting in there and winning this thing." Others speak of the slaughter of innocents, the rape of the land, and the horror of Americana in Southeast Asia. I think we picked a lemon over here. Fact is, though, we're in pretty deep. Back at Fort Bliss and Fort Sam I used to debate with anyone. Here people don't discuss the big picture. They're too preoccupied with their personal problems, job problems, counterpart problems, and getting their mission accomplished.

It strikes me as incongruous and inappropriate, as well as inane, when USO Show people entertain and end up talking about "you brave boys out here, putting your life on the line, suffering for God and Country" and "back home we're with you, God Bless you." Most people here feel uncomfortable hearing this. No one here thinks in those terms.

How should we argue it? That the goal is worthwhile but the price too high? That the goal is not worthwhile, that Communism doesn't threaten me? Or that the price is right if we get first "grabsies" on rubber, tea, coffee, and rice? Problem is this war has passed through so many stages. Our reasons for being here today aren't the same as 5 or 10 years ago. So what's the reason now? LBJ says that we continue to fight now because we're already up to our necks. It's too late to back out.

I've stopped smoking and can't keep my mouth shut (here: hands still). March 16, 8th Field Hospital, Nha Trang. Weight steady at 174.5 lbs. No cigarette in 10 days.

I got lots of advise before coming over. Uncle Morgan advised me never to volunteer. Joe advised me to fight, but for the other side. Mel laughingly coached me on running in a crouch. But the best advice came from a Sgt. who briefed us our 1st day in Saigon. He told us to keep laughing. Tonight I met a chopper pilot, now a patient here. He's been in Vietnam 3 months and is bitter and hostile. I think, either he changes his attitude or his mind will melt before his 12 months are up. You just can't suffer the frustration, rage, disappointments day after day without some perspective.

I awoke from a morning nap to find a hand-made St. Pat's Day card from Maureen Manson, age 12, Troop 201, by my bed. In her note she writes she hopes my day will be fun. And my day turned out pretty good. I'd like to write Maureen a Thank You note but there was no home address.

This respite has given me time to think. I've hit upon a pretty workable program for Lac Thien. I'm thinking of going back. But I'll need 2 good men, a Montagnard interpreter, and a vehicle. Maybe a month out there.

There's a MILPHAP Team here in Nha Trang, capitol of Khanh Hoa Province. I'd like to see how their hospital looks, find out about their mobile program, see how that team is making out. Meanwhile my symptoms are suppressed by donnatal. Last week I discontinued the meds and, WOW! The watery stools and belching and barfing. Stool specimens still negative and other blood work abnormal but non-specific.

Jewish People Are Actually Christians

I regularly find "Jesus Saves" literature on my bed stand. Someone is making rounds while I nap. Today an Army chaplain, a captain, passed out some Easter literature. The title was, "The War Cry" and the cover shows a Roman legionnaire with sword upraised and a look of astonishment. Reflected in his shield is the man he's about to strike, Christ. As the padre delivered the magazine, smiling, I told him I wasn't Christian. He hesitated, then placed the magazine on my bed anyway, with the remark, "Many people say that." My mouth hanging open, he left. I looked at one of the articles in "The War Cry," the one entitled, "The Resurrection—What Proof?"

I probably read it wrong but I had the distinct impression from the evidence it offered that polls which show that people now and in the past believed in the Resurrection of Jesus is the evidence or proof.

Just the other day I told the nurse, a lieutenant, in charge that I didn't want any more religious literature delivered to me, that I was Jewish. The nurse replied that she understood my being Jewish. But, nonetheless, "You're still Christian." I told her that she didn't understand. She went on to console me because Jews must be terribly unhappy because we don't ask God to absolve our sins, unlike Christians who are happy because, despite their sins of all kinds, they can find absolution and be purified. I told her I hadn't the broad catalogue of sins like blasphemy, pride, and not going to Confession. She asked me who came first, myself or my fellow man. I said, myself. Aha, that's a sin, she declared. One's fellow-man must come first. "Of course my fellow-man comes before me," she assured me and gave examples of giving her remaining food, etc. to starving brethren. She's either a liar or a fool, I figured. "O.K., it's you and me here," I began. "No one will rat on you. Give it to me straight. Would you really give your life for some Joe Schlock." She admitted not. A truthful answer. I told her her self-effacing bit was unrealistic, also unnatural. She didn't disagree. For whatever reason she remained insistent that Jews, nonetheless, are Christians and that because Jews don't seek forgiveness for Original Sin we must be miserable, sin-ridden, and guilty.

I'm sure she was unaware how her words, "Jews must be miserable," out of context, can stand as a directive as well as an empathic comment. She probably doesn't know the history that we Jews can't ever forget (and so many Christians can't seem to remember).

Recovering

I'm 175.75 lb. No complaints. Even though my sick-bed ID notes my Jewish religion I continue to get pamphlets about the "life-changing power of Christ." When the registration clerk at the hospital on admission—the ID he generated is on the bed—asked, not my "religion" but my religious "preference," making it sound so casual, so arbitrary, so temporary, I probably should have replied, "I don't know. I like them all."

The novelty of being hospitalized is wearing thin. Must I stay until there is a positive diagnosis?

My friend, Capt. Lou Fishman, the Air Force doctor I'd met last October, visited. He's on his way to Tokyo to play in the Pacific League volleyball championships. He'd just returned from R&R in Hong Kong. Brought me a stack of New York Times and chocolate chip cookies. Answered many of my questions. No other visitors except the chaplain who told me to be at Protestant services at 0900 hours. I give up. I replied, "Yes, Sir."

I wonder if Dr. Don Horsburgh from Pennsylvania has arrived. He's one of our replacements.

He'd written me when he got his assignment to MILPHAP here and was considering bolting for Canada. I didn't blame him. He was not only not an American citizen, he'd already done military service in the Argentine Army. But I'd told him I was learning much and quite satisfied, quite fulfilled, in this place doing this work.

I wonder if the American nurses have arrived. (I'm using the typewriter in the office of the chief of medicine.)

The champ tips the scales at 176 lbs, No symptoms. On no meds. Upper G-I series normal. Fifteen days without a smoke. My nerves are steady. I won 2 chess games.

On American Propaganda, the War and Politicians

A friend of mine, a captain, was featured in an article in the Army Times. In the interview he made it seem like the Open Arms (or Chieu Hoi) Program was a clear success. Why couldn't he say what he used to say over chow at mess in the Bungalow, that his returnees were unhappy living off USAID handouts, that the Government of South VN promises these returnees medical care yet the 14 RVN Army doctors in BMT won't go to their center and treat them. Bill and I still get that chore. (We three American doctors long ago objected as long as those 14 VN doctors enjoyed private practices in town.) The article correctly noted the fact that Darlac Province leads all the others in returnees; most enemy defections take place here.

The Army Times reads like Readers Digest; heros and tear-jerking stories. Once someone printed an article that said RVN soldiers were lazy and chicken and the shit hit the fan. Someone once wrote that Saigon was a big brothel. Again, shit hit the fan. Yet every GI here knows that Saigon is about graft and black market; just walk down the streets and see the jeep parts for sale, C-rations and "gifts" from people in the USA marked "NOT FOR SALE" for sale.

Sitting at the mess table you hear stories about the average RVN soldier being under-trained and poorly led. There are exceptions but I'm talking about guys who fought alongside them, who watched their officers in briefing session, whose fatigue uniforms were tailored skin tight.

The pacification angle is being overworked. I mentioned the Revolutionary Development Corps, those young VN being trained in home economics and agriculture, etc. and who wear black pajamas and live in hamlets so to beat the V.C. at their own game. I've had time to work with these kids. They're in over their heads. They don't know anything about government policy even as they represent the government at the hamlet level.

*I read we should stop the bombing of the North because it's **not** effective; the flow of men and arms southward continues at an all time high. I read we should stop the bombing of the North because it **is** effective as it diverts labor to repairing damage, creating shortages of vital materials, and destroys the concept of "sanctuary." Who will the GOP nominate to run in 1968? No doubt, LBJ. RFK has his idea but doesn't know what he's talking about. (And Reagan says, "get in there and win with whatever it takes." Win what? He, too, doesn't know what he's talking about.) It could be a cheaper war if we stopped the black market and profiteering, the theft and robbery, the graft and payola.*

This war isn't for territory or killing people. It's a contest for men's minds. We're good at that. We've got the tradition and machinery in Hollywood and Madison Avenue. But, excuse the line from Music Man, "You've got to know the territory!" We don't know the "territory."

All this talk about "feelers," "signals," "signs" from Hanoi. The cartoon of LBJ waiting for the signal from Hanoi. Like a seance. Hanoi has been answering us all along. The answer is, no.

The Military, Homosexuality and One Doctor's Dilemma

Met an interesting fellow in the mess hall, a doctor. He's a patient here on the psychiatric ward and he's going into psychiatry. He told me his story. A week ago he woke up at night to find his tent-mates, one a major, the other a captain, engaged in a homosexual contact. This is a legal matter. My friend subsequently sought advice from a friend. If he reports these doctors it's his word against theirs and they could make it tough on him. On the advice of a friend he went to his CO and submitted a formal report of what he'd seen. Then, in the event that his credibility was questioned (i.e., that the major might accuse him of hallucinating), he took himself to the 8th Field Hospital for a psychiatric evaluation and clearance. The staff here treat him like any other patient. On rounds he must stand at parade rest at the foot of his bed like the rest. He must ask permission to leave, walk around, etc. There is a mental patient in his outfit that he'd been treating who is now, here, on the same ward with him at the 8th Field Hospital. The nurses write in their reports, "withdrawn." He'd eat at the officer's table in the mess but never speak. Imagine what it's like for him. Now he talks and talks. To me. Never spoke at mealtime out of fear he'd be asked what ward he was on or what his disease was.

Anyhow, he wanted to do what was right by the army but turning in your superior officer as a homosexual isn't easy. And neither is being admitted for a psychiatric work-up with no exception for being a physician or because of the nature of his admission. (By now you know my opinion of the psychiatrists here.) So I commiserate with this fellow and wonder how it all will turn out. Surely he won't return to his outfit, not while those two are there. Of course, there's always the possibility he's putting me on; really is disturbed. I considered this. But I believe him.

Last Days in Nha Trang

Reality as metaphor: They never identified an organism to account for my gasto-enteritis. I simply recovered enough and then asked to be discharged. Looking back I'm struck by this irony: an American is brought low by an invisible enemy, very small, a local. Nobody could find and catch the bugger despite repeated searches. To me, this summary works equally well as a military summary and a medical summary. The difference: *they* (the military) kept plugging, I called it quits and left.

I'm leaving. You won't hear from me until I reach Ban Me Thuot. If there's trouble getting a flight out I'll stay in Jose Segarra's quarters; he's my doctor here and he leaves for Tokyo tomorrow.

I wanted to leave the 8th Field Hospital early last Friday because I had a seat on a plane to BMT but the administrative office made me wait until 10:00, a rule, so I missed the flight. I was obliged to go to Camp McDermott, actually a cluster of tents not far down the beach, where I'd be put up until a flight could be arranged. I sat around and chatted with VN cleaning ladies. Because of my rank they spared me the tent; said I could wait in a French hotel instead, also on the beach but nearer the center of town.

My flight was reserved for Saturday morning so the driver took me to this hotel, actually 5 rooms at ground level. The rest is restaurant, outdoor patio cafe, bar. And who was eating there with 2 Air Force doctors and 2 beautiful VN girls but Lou Fishman! His volleyball tournament in Tokyo was cancelled by MACV. "There's a war going on and we can't sponsor a volleyball game in Japan." (Funny he should mention that because a MACV golf team just left for a tournament in Thailand.) So I left my hotel room and moved into Lou's villa and that night we went on the town together. Nha Trang used to be an R&R Center so there's a surplus of clubs, bars, girls of all prices. We spent a long time talking before hitting the sack.

R&R in Hong Kong

I took R&R (Rest and Recuperation) with Lt. Brown. On arrival in Hong Kong, Hank and I had first to deal with the many girls who, at the airport, offered to be our mistresses, living with us, etc. Hank and I had shopping on our minds, not schtupping. For me it was all about having clothes tailored (which I never wore because, once home and married and having recovered all that lost weight, nothing fit) and shopping in Kowloon for gifts in preparation for family reunions and the wedding. But I did think to try something totally different and out of character for me. I had a manicure. Why not? No one was looking who knew me. The Chinese girl rounded out my nails so my large hands with broad fingers looked weird. I don't know what she was thinking. The Thai dessert set I bought has never seen use. The lady's beggar beads were worn just once. And the carved ivory chess set was never set out on a board. So I regret not having taking the Bangkok option instead of Hong Kong for R&R. I regret not going there and buying one of those huge, marvelous "fornicating elephants" wood carvings I'd heard so much about. I like conversation, and that would have made a singular conversation-starter for the living room in whatever apartment we found. (Or conversation-stopper.)

> I remember that we had a wonderful time together. After we arrived in Hong Kong what you wanted most was a long, hot shower, and then a pedicure. I really teased you about having a manicure. But, now that I look back, it sounds quite logical to me. I think I took a shower and then quickly followed that by heading for an ice-cream parlor. Ice-cream was then, and remains now, my dessert passion. Of course in South Vietnam we were deprived of real ice-cream. Everything we were served called ice-cream there was made of powder. I really hated the stuff! As a result my craving for real ice-cream by the time we'd landed in Hong Kong was at an all time peak. We both had ice-cream. Then, off to shopping we both went [Hank Brown, personal communication].

I Return to Ban Me Thuot

Action continues in Darlac Sector. Buon Ho was hit again and an American advisor from the Bungalow killed in an ambush a week later. Hamlets around Ban Me Thuot have been mortared. South Vietnamese soldiers fired upon the Montagnard strikers at the Ban Don camp. Next week Dr. Niem meets with representatives of all the district dispensaries to discuss medical care in the districts. (They have been meeting regularly all year.)

MILPHAP doctors run the Ban Me Thuot civilian hospital, provide actual patient care. The new American chief nurse and the VN chief nurse met to discuss the incoming 5 American nurses. No member of the MILPHAP Team was invited to attend this meeting. Stan stopped the American chief nurse before she left for Saigon and in the brief time he had with her tried to straighten her out. She was saying that her records showed 19 technicians at the hospital working now. Stan objected, telling her that wasn't true, that he wouldn't lie over something like this, and to please forget what they were telling her in Saigon. She could check for herself. There were 9, not 19, technicians at the hospital of which 2 had transferred away and 2 were currently ill, leaving 5. So 5 American nurses are coming. To do what, teach? Teach whom? When? What would they teach? Stan put these questions to the woman. The program she is planning to initiate is evidently unstructured and ill-defined and based on out-of-date statistics.

Doctor Niem is in favor of my suggestion that a government dispensary be built and staffed at Ban Don.

Replacements for our Team are coming in, Pfcs. 47 days left. It's unusual not to have orders by this time; usually they're sent out 2 months prior to departure. A lot of people here are sitting on their hands. Their counterparts who they're supposed to advise don't like, trust, or respect them. They spend the year faking it.

One of our replacements, a Sgt. has arrived and, although assigned to MILPHAP, his specific orders don't mention that. So, after a week here at the Bungalow, nobody is sure where he fits, who has authority over him. Officially he's not assigned to MILPHAP.

I take Stan's ward when he holds sick call at the missionary's dispensary. But our mission here isn't to support the Christian missionaries, to put their dispensary in competition with the province hospital. Stan knows how I feel but can't say no to these people.

Rains have begun, heavy downpour in late afternoon and again at night. It's cooling and refreshing but the insects and mosquitoes seem to be everywhere. I expect malaria will be on the rise again.

22 days without a cigarette.

I've no immediate plans for mobile trips. The enemy is raising hell throughout the Sector and the MILPHAP mission makes sense only in political terms. I'm not going to think about it for a while.

One officer and 5 enlisted men have gonorrhea and all name the same woman as contact, an American girl, an International Volunteer here to teach sewing. (Her reputation began to suffer the moment she made known that she carried condoms with her.)

We cure sick people. That little boy with beri-beri is ready to play soccer. The woman with the goiter had it removed. The little boy with terribly swollen and raw, infected face, who'd been courageously coming for treatment since last September—we're trying a new skin ointment AMCE Alumni sent and the skin is healing! We snatched a little Montagnard girl with fulminant tetanus from death's door. There's been only one death on Stan's ward this month!

My technicians in outpatient clinic are eager students and I continue to learn from them. The VN general in charge of II Corps Area inspects the hospital next week. The place has been a bee hive of activity, fresh paint for everything, beds, walls, tables. Offices and passageways are scrubbed clean. Handymen are pruning the trees and landscaping the grounds.

I received your box of kosher salami and it was covered with fungus and mold. I cleaned it off, peeling the outer skin. The meat was great but we have to eat it quickly or mold will re-form, even in the refrigerator.

Dr. Don Horsborgh has arrived. He came to the states last year (Pennsylvania) to intern and married an American girl. His visa expired and he was drafted. Now he is in Vietnam. Our new Project Vietnam doctor, a surgeon, is Dr. John Ballou. One of my two counterparts, the VN lady doctor, left for the Delta to be with her husband.

Stan had two children, a brother and sister, on his ward with pneumonia. The boy was doing pretty well. Late one night his mother complained that he wasn't sleeping so the night technician [inappropriately] gave him 100 mg of phenobarbital and the boy died. The next morning Dr. Niem came to talk to the distraught parents and told them he'd died because he hadn't received enough antibiotics. The unhappy parents left with the daughter.

Interesting slang: USA is the "Land of the Big PX." Being close to the end of your tour in Vietnam is being "Short." The point at which a GI has to stop sexual activities and the accompanying risk of catching a venereal disease and bringing it home to his wife is, "P.C.O.D." (Pussy Cut Off Date). Viet Cong soldiers are "Charlie." It's all the same is, "Same-Same." Hurryup is, "Di Di Mao"

An Epidemic of Violent Deaths

A Montagnard striker (or "Trong San" soldier) came in from Lam Dong province suffering belly pain with cramps. He was also, for the past hour, losing his vision. He told of drinking rum the day before. It sounded like the poisonings that have been occurring in Buon Ho and Lac Thien. (He died an hour later.) Such a thing, I was told, was without precedent. Reports of methyl alcohol poisonings were coming out of Saigon, as well. This seemed terribly suspicious. Was it deliberate? So far it's not in the papers.

There have been, in recent weeks, sudden outbreaks of violent illness and death in the Central Highlands and no one knows the cause. Initially it seemed unstoppable as it spread. Lac Thien was first hit with 26 deaths. By the time the epidemic was traced to methyl alcohol poisoning from home-made alcohol from stills here in BMT, the V.C. had been accused of poisoning wells and Montagnards had held enough sacrifices and parties over their sick and dying to pass around that bad alcohol. Thus the high toll. Next it happened in Di Lin and Bao Lac. The night before last we were notified that Buon Ho was involved; the villages Cung Kiem, Dat Hieu, and Buon Tring. (I had taken my medical patrol there in December, treated people and immunized against cholera and plague.) Dr. Niem asked me to fly to Lac Thien. I had asked that Y Rulick, the medicine chief at the Lac Thien dispensary, come to BMT for 2 months further training. Now I asked that Y Rulick come along with me plus two Vietnamese public health workers.

It was rough work, trying to confirm deaths, interview family, question and examine everyone reporting in sick, separating the frightened from the poisoned. Was there a poisoning? What was rumor and what fact? I was confined to the Buon Ho dispensary because, since my last mobile trip out here and the attacks by North VN troops, these 3 villages involved fell under V.C. control so I couldn't track down all the leads. And the District HQ, the compound where I'd stayed, guarded by RF-PF plus American advisors, wasn't able to provide armed escort for me. They felt the V.C. may have deliberately poisoned the people and that they may have done this to confuse us and make us send soldiers here and there and leave the compound vulnerable to attack.

I got enough data for a preliminary report and a chopper flew me out that same evening. My Vietnamese and Montagnard counterparts remained there to continue the investigation. Dr. Niem is II Corps public health director and he is expecting more outbreaks. Is it methyl alcohol? If so, has it been deliberate? I was asked for advice on how to treat this so a directive could be sent to other province health officials. Dr. Niem and I agreed that not all the deaths had, in fact, been confirmed and of those that were confirmed, did they die of the same cause? Because of the hysteria that follows scares like this you can't simply treat everyone with the same drugs. Someone must determine who is sick and who is not, and of the sick, who is suspected of poisoning and who isn't.

Buon Ho District needs 9 investigators including 3 doctors working steadily for 3 days to cope with their reported epidemic. They send me and 3 counterparts. And I was removed that same night. I work for Dr. Niem. He'll do what he thinks best. Already reports from Phan Thiet have turned out to be cholera, a problem best directed by Americans and handled by Vietnamese. The hundreds of interviews which must be conducted must be conducted without language barrier, which was why I didn't object to being pulled out of Buon Ho. I had no interpreter. How was I to take a medical history, to know when the patient first fell ill and see if there was a relationship with a meal. Peasants don't wear watches, don't have clocks.

Case of the Woman with the Hole in Her Face: The Look of Corruption (Ours)

I met the major, a dentist and maxillo-facial surgeon, at the 8th Field Hospital when I was hospitalized there. He told me he specialized in facial reconstruction and was interested in carcinomas of the face. He believes it's caused by betel-nut chewing (the paste used is a lime-mixture). I had told him about a Montagnard patient, the wife of a hospital employee, at Ban Me Thuot. Half her face is gone, probably carcinoma. A long shot is Yaws or one of the destructive fungal diseases. The hole through her cheek is wide. I told her husband that there was no cure but he begged me to look for a specialist. I insisted there was no hope but agreed to inquire. Were any surgeons interested? The major was. He was working on a hypothesis that squamous cell carcinoma is related to chewing betel nut, a common practice here. He said his staff would take good care of her if she came. I told him we'd be grateful for anything he would do or suggest for the patient. So I'll send the patient to him soon as I get home. He'll take photos, take the history, and do a biopsy. Cancer or not, the lady is beyond surgery, radiotherapy, or drug cure. I told the patient's husband to tell the family to stand-by.

There was no provision for her husband to accompany her or for an interpreter. I was reassured by the major that his staff would take good care of her. The final 4 weeks were trying to get a flight. We had many false alarms, rushing out in ambulance, waiting at the airstrip. Pilots were watching for planes going to Nha Trang to let me know on a moments notice. A Vietnamese ambulance driver was ready to race to the village and get the patient. The last 3 days I was in daily contact either with the major or his staff at the 8th Field Hospital in Nha Trang telling them to "stand by."

I'd first met the woman, H Yak M'lo (Hu-yuk-mello), age 45, at the urging of her husband. She lay in her longhouse, very, very frightened. Half her face looked eaten away. I learned she had never been away from her village, she understood no language other than Rhade, and she cannot speak because of the facial damage. For three years she has been fed and nursed by her sons and daughters. In their longhouse she sleeps in the room that serves as living and dining room. That's where there is a fireplace. The floor, of bamboo strips, is easy to sweep. Of everything that falls through the cracks, the animals below, the pigs, goats, cows, check and eat the garbage. Although invalid, she was at the center of her family's life.

She had wanted to go to Nha Trang and be examined despite being assured there would be no treatment. I couldn't refuse. So when I had recovered my own health and returned to BMT I contacted her husband. He wanted this. I remember waiting for the med-evac helicopter to pick her up. She lay on a stretcher. Her eldest son was there to see her off. I decided I'd go along and stay in Nha Trang as long as possible to help look after her. I told her son to tell her to look at my face and remember it. Once in Nha Trang, full of so many Vietnamese and Americans, she'd be in a sea of total strangers. It was important she know me by sight.

On the helicopter, as it lifted off, she took my hand which I held firmly until she fell asleep. She was scared. An hour later we set down at the Emergency Room of the 8th Field Hospital. Rotors still going we ducked low and carried H Yak inside. I called the major and he came to look at her. He paused, then said, as if there had been the possibility of his rejecting her (which both alarmed and offended me): "We'll take her."

H Yak was more than fortunate to be admitted to the 8th Field Hospital with its lights, air-conditioning, private rooms, 24 hour-a-day nurses, TV and radio. I went to stay with an Air Force buddy and visited her daily. She was grossly iron deficient. I wrote a note to the major asking that he provide dextrose and water intravenously with vitamins. She looked worse and worse; she had given up. She was homesick and looked terrible. She no longer opened her eyes to look at me, didn't seem to recognize me. If she died here how could I go back and face her family? But how to give her encouragement? Her doctor said she'd be discharged in 4 days so that was good news. The studies and teaching would be completed. But how to tell her? How to find someone who spoke Rhade. I knew American Special Forces wounded were patients here so maybe a wounded Rhade striker was here, too. I heard of such a patient and went to find him.

When I found this Montagnard I simply showed him my brass bracelets, presented to me by Rhade tribesmen at Lac Thien. I spoke the Rhade greeting. We both knew some Vietnamese so I told him about H Yak and asked him to visit her. He gestured to his cast—he was wounded in the leg and couldn't move. I next asked him to teach me to say, in Rhade, "Be of good cheer; you leave for home in 4 days." He taught and I practiced, rehearsed. (It must have seemed odd to the American GIs in the next beds watching TV.) I finally got it down enough and hurried to H Yak's side to tell her. I said it over and over. She never opened her eyes. She never moved.

The major told me she had incurable cancer and gave me some advice for making her comfortable, feeding her. I had to return to BMT ahead of her. On the day promised a chopper brought her to BMT and an American medic picked her up at the helipad and took her to the BMT hospital and I was there. The first person to reach her was a Rhade nurse who took her hand and spoke their greeting. By the time I reached the stretcher I could hear the sobbing and crying, the weak voice of this woman who had come home at last. But the sounds were coming from under the bandage over the left side of her head. Her lips never moved because she only had half a face.

H Yak, helpless and dying, showed all of us that America, with all its planes, TVs and, yes, medical drugs, doesn't compare to her family, even if her life depended on it.

When her husband asked me for the doctors report, his findings and recommendations I pulled the note he had pinned to her. "Case Summary: 20 year history betel nut chewing in Montagnard, 3 year history possible cancer, Path. Dx: Squamous Cell Carcinoma. Recommendations: dressing should be with petrolatum gauze instead of cotton. Provide irrigating syringe for feedings. Change dressings daily.

I went begging for petrolatum gauze at the Special Forces compound in BMT and put in a requisition for the syringe through our supply channels.

The major got his biopsy and research case and I got to feel like his chump. His agreeing to see my patient at the hospital hadn't been offered with her his in-patient; he'd meant he'd peek at her outside the hospital door and there decide if she met his research requirements. But the deal he'd struck with me was that he'd provide at least, in exchange, a minimally caring experience.

Follow-up: I wish the major had provided the medical items he'd recommended. He'd had them on hand. I wish his staff hadn't taken away H Yak's blanket. They'd kept it; a dime a dozen for a GI but representing real work, time, and savings for a Montagnard. A replacement blanket would have been an adequate gesture in return for a rare, unique research case. I wish they'd have given her the intravenous with iron and vitamins that I'd requested so that, in her last weeks when she was passing, she might have been more present and more connected with her suffering family. On May 2, shortly after H Yak's return home, I wrote the nurse at the hospital who'd taken care of me when I'd been a patient there (and lectured me on Christian charity) and asked if she'd look for this patient's blanket and return it to me, or else grab any white replacement blanket and toss it onto the next med-evac chopper from BMT and write my name on it. H Yak died at 3:00 p.m., May 21. Her husband came to tell me. It was as if the major had lost somehow sight of the trees for the forest. And the forest was his personal forest. In any event I was sorry I'd sent her to the major at the Eighth Field Hospital in Nha Trang. I never got that blanket.

Ban Me Thuot Sound Bites

The Bungalow laundry hasn't been operating for several weeks. I've received no clean laundry since 10 April [letter written April 30] *so I've been wearing my black pajamas for the past 2 days. Everybody has to make a remark, a common one being, "V.C.! V.C.!" to which I put up my hands and say, "Chieu Hoi" (which means I've surrendered to the government side).*

I'm sitting in the dispensary at the Bungalow in Capt. Naylor's office. I sneaked a peak into a folder on the desk and read a copy of a letter written by the senior advisor here recommending Capt. Naylor [the new MACV doctor we'd nicknamed "Howdy-Doody"] *for a position with another Advisory Team. The Col. credits him with the VD Program in town (that's our MILPHAP program) and for personally investigating and treating the methyl alcohol poisoning in Buon Ho. (I went, not Naylor), and so on. I think he wants to get rid of Capt. Naylor.*

About parades and "peaceniks," few people here take such sentiment seriously. Same with "peaceniks." All that really bothers very few over here.

The American nurses have arrived, three of them. They're civilians and nobody is sure what they're supposed to do.

A Vietnamese fortune-teller, former patient of mine, has had me for dinner several times. Hoan tells me it's because I'm likable. They've treated me well, as an honored guest. My fortune was read last week after dinner. Mr. Hy asked me when I'd be returning to Vietnam, asked as a serious and common question. (Stan was recently asked the same thing when interviewed by a radio announcer. His reply was: "I don't expect to come back." It seemed to offend.) My guarded response to Mr. Hy, my friend, was that, should I return, it wouldn't be as a soldier. I'd come as a traveler visiting friends.

Things are quiet now but 101st Airborne people are appearing around here. One 101st Division major came doing a survey. Easy questions to answer. My evaluation of the Medical Field Service School at Fort Sam Houston? "Waste of time." Would I consider Army for a career? "Never."

I'm eager to discontinue mobile trips. G-2 (Intelligence) estimates several North Vietnam Divisions around Ban Me Thuot now. If and when they pounce I want to be home.

Two Pfc. replacements came. They have had no preparation at Fort Sam, no background for this mission or this country, weren't issued any equipment (no weapons, no canteen, no sleeping bag) and didn't have an in-country briefing. They speak English and are very nervous.

More replacements, all Pfcs. Hospitals and dispensaries desperately short on supplies and trained personnel and we offer young, untrained, and scared GIs in over their heads, albeit briefed about their superiority by virtue of being American. I remember those briefings. "Any American high school student knows more about medicine and hygiene than a Vietnamese nurse or technician!"

Reflections: During that breached delivery I wrote about above, when the health worker had asked me to correct the fetus' position I told him I had neither witnessed nor performed such a procedure. My clinical experience on Ob-Gyn had been just 3 months' rotation as an intern. But when I demurred to attempt the procedure, an external cephalic version, the health worker urged me to and the woman did, too; she really didn't want to go to the hospital. What I did was go through the motions, doing little other than confirming the buttocks first presentation, and then sent for a chopper. (A healthy delivery of a first born. I never learned whether delivery was by Caesarian or vaginal delivery following a successful external version, or just a lucky breech birth. But, I learned, her joy was indescribable.)

Take-home lesson: Briefing and bluster aren't the same thing, just as being fully informed and being full of yourself aren't. Just because you're American and a GI doesn't mean you're fit to do a job. I'm reminded here of an anecdote a friend and teacher here in Massachusetts recently told me, a story that makes one smile and wince at the same time. He recently asked his college class — he teaches religion — to give their opinion as to from what continent the next pope would be chosen (the Vatican is deliberating this matter as I write these lines). One student raised his hand. "What's a 'continent'?"

Back to Quang Nhieu and a Canard Waiting to Erupt

I went back to Quang Nhieu, the Regional-Popular Forces compound at the Mewal Coffee Plantation last week with Hoan and Pfc. Aragon because of more reports of poisonings and 16 deaths, all Vietnamese. Several sick, one's survived. Wood alcohol again. Two days ago 6 Montagnards from Buon Pak came in with the symptoms. They reported 2 deaths in their village. I made my reports. The rest is up to Dr. Niem and the police. No one is tracing the source of the hootch or impounding bottles. Seems they're waiting for laboratory confirmation from Saigon. My trip to Quang Nhieu was by helicopter; I refused to go by road. It was good to see friends at the RFPF compound where I stayed some time ago. They invited me to stick around a few days and fight the V.C. Interesting, as many Vietnamese have died as have Montagnards from the bad alcohol yet rumors are spreading among the Montagnards that the VN are intentionally poisoning them. The Psychological Warfare people haven't yet taken action.

"Banish," "Floxie" and "Claymore": Sweet Sorrow, June 1967

We had our final [MACV] meeting day. A general gave a farewell speech mentioning our unpublicized mission — that only Fort Sam and several people in Washington know about us — we'll receive no publicity. But it's the most important assignment over here.

Stan left early this morning. Still no orders or port call for me. There was a ceremony attended by the province chief and notables, VN and American, and the MILPHAP Team was presented certificates of appreciation. Then a farewell dinner at the Bungalow. Big party in our room. Bill leaves next week. All the enlisted men go home the 19th. I wait. Perhaps, in its infinite wisdom and in terms of a big picture and the greater need, the army is doing what must be done. Funny thing. When the province chief presented us with our certificates, the interpreter translated Banach, Baxley, and Climo as "Banish," "Floxie," and "Claymore," so that's a little joke among ourselves.

My brother writes me an advisory: "About your not receiving termination orders and date, unlike your military confreres, this, coupled with recent newscasts of Secretary NcNamara's urgent request to extend everyone's tour within the next thirty days, has stirred quite a bit of emotion."

My checking reveals that my file, for some reason, is sidelined onto the desk at MACV Headquarters. The people who cut these orders need that file. I'm informally advised that I leave Vietnam the 11th of this month. The source is official. I expect I'll fly to Saigon, verify, and then be on my way home Sunday.

I did and was.

12

This Story's Coda

Winning Hearts and Minds:
The Rest of That Story

Off duty, on our own, being ourselves, there appeared one-to-one connections that probably were closer to the heart of our mission than those that went into our monthly reports. There was less "white noise," so to speak, in those spontaneous and informal interpersonal relationships. I'm referring, for example, to John Guingrich being approached by a Vietnamese mother who'd heard of him, his ways and manner and Christian values, and proposing that he marry her daughter.[1] I'm thinking, too, of Daniel Melberg, who was asked by his colleague in the hospital lab, a Rhade technician, Y Suah Buon Krong, with whom he'd developed a friendship, for help with his English lessons.[2] And Bill Baxley, who was asked by his nurse if he'd be her surrogate parent. And Hank Brown, who worked in Dr. Niem's office, where Niem's secretary, Co Hoa, who loved to sing, was so fond of Hank. And Stan Banach, who held sick-call for those seeking treatment at the missionary infirmary wherein he was able, without obstruction, to be the healer he was capable of being. Or Al Rodriguez, whose compassion for the villager whose very sick child died shortly after admission prompted him to buy a little casket and arrange a ride in a helicopter that was flying near his home area. Here is another Rodriguez story in his own words:

> I used to buy as much meat as I could at the market and veggies and mushrooms and would spend my time at Buon Le "A." Meals were usually prepared by H Nhe and her mother while her husband and I talked. Guests would come over and eat. Her father, Y Chal, worked at the warehouse where supplies were kept between the hospital and the administration

203

building. Sundays I would attend Mass in Rhade and French at the Church about ½ mile to right of hospital if you were facing it. I spent all my spare time there, took many people there. I used to take the crew to celebrations that I was invited to by my Ede friends in Boun Le "A," Buon Le "B," Buon Ea Nao, Buon Kotan. I talked a lot, listened, went hunting with them behind Buon Le "A." I used my weapon to kill lizards also. My mother sent me pinto beans and I taught them how to plant and eat them. We found lemon grass. I taught them to eat cactus like we did. Used to borrow big trucks from Special Forces camp and take Rhade to harvest bamboo a couple of miles north of the power plant. Hung out with many FULRO. Always wondered if I was on somebody's list [personal communication].

About Five Elephants in the Room:
Politics, Personalities, Customs, Systems and Corruption

We were doctors trained in the arts of healing. We weren't politicians or diplomats. To prepare for our civic action mission we took many different courses prior to coming to Vietnam and had many orientation lectures once in-country. But no course or lecture and no teacher or lecturer ever mentioned, let alone explained or prepared us for, what we would really be fussing over, five elephants that would be waiting for us in our consultation rooms, a presence that would squeeze us and crowd us, that would frustrate and repeatedly derail us, and would ultimately corrupt us. Traditions and politics, ours and theirs, secrete an invisible force field of expectation, power, obligation, and secrets. System differences inevitably feels like personality differences, and the real, and ubiquitous, personality issues, ours and theirs, always have their own agendas, usually so obscure that the person, him or herself, doesn't even know their workings let alone sees their presence. The fifth elephant that our leaders and teachers, like our politicians and diplomats, knew well and even fretted about themselves only never saw fit to give us a heads-up about, was corruption and the many types of integrity failure that term embraces. They could have alerted us to this, to our own corruptions if not to theirs. Young doctors, fresh from training, idealists, are not naturals at gaming a system. (One wonders about that MILPHAP doctor who was dismissed at the start of his assignment for subordination, or the one requiring psychiatric attention during his tour, or that entire MILPHAP team that was rejected by the chief of medicine. Were these casualties of this reality? Was General Humphries' alleged lack of faith in our mission — the rumor that he didn't "believe" in it — his own candid reaction to this reality?)

So, in our own ways and in our own time, we became corrupted ourselves. How could it be otherwise? We thought about and attended to and retreated to our idiosyncratic needs, habits, and biases, our own personal priorities, in the face of intractable and insolvable problems. But here's the irony. It was at this level, looking after ourselves and our own agendas, that we most genuinely and sincerely came to win over hearts and minds. And let our own hearts and minds be won over to the suffering and cause of individual Vietnamese, highlander and lowlander, who we'd let ourselves become close to, a closeness that was reciprocated. In other words, unofficially and off the record and not at all on our MILPHAP to-do list, our "corrupted" hearts and minds seemed not to have stopped tuning in, reaching out, and connecting.

There's an uncanny parallel between a personal experience in Vietnam like mine, how I got in and got out, and our nation's experience of getting in and getting out, that seems appropriate to point out. First, when I got into all this it was because circumstances made it happen. That's why I'd felt led into it, manipulated into it; I didn't seek it. Second, my being called up might have been avoided in the first place had I paid closer attention to details. Third, when, at last I was inescapably involved, my sense of duty kicked in. Fourth, there were complex agendas that involved my being disingenuous and not entirely forthcoming in what I said and did to manage my mission. Finally, my getting out became something of a cliff-hanger. The concern was I'd stay longer than I had to. And when I left I had no desire to go back. Does this not parallel the larger American involvement?

Many Vietnamese expected Americans to return if things got really bad, just as we had, in a sense, primed them to expect. Thus, according to some sources, when the North launched their final assault and came crashing across the central highlands (just as North Vietnam's General Vo Nguyen Giap, architect of the victory at Dien Bien Phu, had done years before) there seemed to be an expectation, especially with the American Seventh Fleet offshore, that we'd return. Instead, we evacuated our people and selected allies. Saigon surrendered without a fight. We were done there. When it came time to ratify the Ceasefire Agreement the Senate ignored it. We'd already moved on.

About my mission, it seems we failed. We didn't win enough Vietnamese hearts and minds for them to give enough support to their government during that period of intense Vietcong insurgency (just as, on the other side of the ocean, we didn't win enough American hearts and minds over to supporting what our *own* government had been doing at that time in the face of what might be looked at as our *own* anti-war "insurgency"). But, on a person-to-person level, as individuals, I believe, we of MILPHAP did help people, and they appreciated this; this is what became my permanent memory. If the hearts and minds that were actually redirected were ours to them and theirs to us, *as individuals,* then this was an unintended consequence. And if, in this, there was left behind in Vietnam a cadre of Vietnamese people, highland and lowland, who felt affection for American people and whose memories and feelings served to blunt any nationwide rancor towards us in the years that followed our withdrawal, that, too, was an unintended consequence. But I embrace those unintended consequences. Just being there as a visitor, a tourist, I came to a new appreciation of that feeling one has simply knowing that someone who has mattered to you remembers you. And asks about you.

My outpatient clinic VN technician told me that wherever he goes in and around Ban Me Thuot and among people he meets from the districts, they all ask him if he knows "Dr. Climo." People remember and ask about me.

13

Returning Home and Moving On, Then Going Back

I slipped home, unnoticed, to anti-war rallies and Black Panthers. I married, began my years of specialty training in psychiatry at Yale and then the Austen Riggs Center in Massachusetts, and then took up practice. We started our family. (That's the short version.) The longer version for those years, 1967–75, would include my pausing to look up at a television screen while on evening rounds as a first-year resident at the West Haven VA Hospital to see scenes of Ban Me Thuot under attack during the 1968 TET Offensive and my immediately writing to the 734th Medical Detachment mailing address in Ban Mc Thuot for information. (A MILPHAP captain's response is reprinted in Appendix III.) The longer version would include my traveling to Washington, D.C., to protest America's incursion into Cambodia, my giving talks to doctors about tropical medicine, and my wife and me buying an old, three-story Victorian house in Pittsfield, Massachusetts, that ensured plenty of rooms to grow into including a 3rd floor apartment with its own bath. There was ample wall space, for example, for my Montagnard crossbows and ax, and shelf space for my Rhade *ding nam*, that wind-instrument of reeds extending from a gourd, and woven Rhade basket and memorabilia and books about Vietnam, as well a second entrance and private office for seeing private patients. That longer version would certainly highlight one very unexpected but most welcome telephone call.

In 1975 Nguyen Hoan and his wife Tran Thi Kim Sa came to live with us. The story of their escape from Vietnam and how they found and contacted me is recounted in the two feature stories by journalist, Kirk Scharfenberg, "Vietnamese refugee couple coming to city" and "A telegram opened the door in escaping from Vietnam," that appeared in the Berkshire Eagle in June 1975 and are reproduced in the Appendix I and II.) It was in Pittsfield, Massachusetts, that I went from being "Doctor Climo" to "Larry" and where the Hoans, adopting his last name as their family name, had their first child, a son. Hoan hadn't yet begun having the dreams that survivors of trauma have when they begin remembering those left behind, those not so lucky, those who didn't make it out.

Hoan had since become an Air Force pilot, but now with so many out-of-work pilots in America unable to find work, he found a position in the mail room of a local mail-order business. This proved not only an adequate source of income for the couple but companionship for me as well, inasmuch as the hospital where I was now on staff, the Austen Riggs Center in Stockbridge, was across the street from his new workplace, Country Curtains by the Red Lion Inn. So, driving to and from work each day Hoan and I got to talk about adjusting to life in America, family, politics, work, and just nothing — just enjoying being on the road together. In time, our local friends, Larry and Abby Pratt in Great Barrington, aware this young Vietnamese family had never had or lived in a place of their own, offered a free-standing and fully furnished artist's cottage on their property at a rent that the Hoans could afford.

It was a bittersweet parting when Hoan and Sa and their son, Lawrence ("Little Larry") left to move to California to be reunited with Sa's large family, which had been sponsored by a church group out of their refugee camp, and restart their American experience amongst a rapidly expanding Vietnamese refugee community outside Los Angeles. But we agreed to stay in touch.

Once I began writing this book in the fall of 2012 I took a break and actually did return to Vietnam, this time as a visitor and this time with my wife, Diane, who had always wanted to see for herself those places I'd written to her about so many years before. This was to be a private tour, just for the two of us. The Central Highlands, not really open to tourists because of anti-government agitations there, had only recently become more accessible and, while it was still not on many people's list of places to visit, it was very much at the top of ours.

Returning to Vietnam as a Tourist: Novelty, Disparity, Detachment and Something Else

People ask me what it was like, going back to Vietnam, to Communist Vietnam, returning as a visitor, on a tour that took us from Hanoi (and an overnight cruise in Halong Bay) in the north through Hue and Hoi An, Nha

Trang and Danang in the central part, and into the Central Highlands to Ban Me Thuot (now Buon Ma Thout), Buon Ho, and Ban Don, and finally to Saigon (Ho Chi Minh City), and then on a boat trip into the Mekong Delta to Hoa Binh Phuoc. It was all, for the most part, a novelty. Everything was new, exciting, and different. Nothing was as I remembered it.

What impressed me the most? The disparities, the contrasts, such as between used and new, primitive and modern, neglected and indulged, patched-together versus cranes erecting contemporary skyscrapers, poor versus wealthy (referring to both places and people). There wasn't much in between. It was as if, rather than update and refine legislation with the changing times, the government was content to keep existing laws as they were and simply enforce them selectively, as if to ensure that anyone and everyone, at one time or another, was doing something illegal and, therefore, to my cynical thinking, obliged to pay a bribe to someone simply to remain in business.

How did I feel? Mostly detached. There were no points of personal connection. Without realizing it at the time, I had hoped someone would remember me or my mission.

There were three exceptions. One was my unexpected feeling of closeness to our young Rhade guide, Y Sam, in Ban Me Thuot. Why? (I wondered about that the whole time we were in BMT.) Was it because he was named for Samuel of the Bible (he'd told us), like my own father, Samuel Climo? Was it because of what he'd whispered in my ear when he saw I was struggling to complete the obligatory cup of rice wine while drinking together through separate straws with the head of the house in the Rhade longhouse where we were guests? (When I looked up at him, pleading, and mouthed, "I can't do this," he leaned down and whispered, "Just pretend to drink.") Or was it his taking us to where the Bungalow used to be before it was burned down due to an electric fire (or so some said), pointing out where the soccer field across the road had since been expanded to incorporate those grounds, and taking us to where the original market stood? (Dr. Niem's house, like the missionary compound — even the 155th Aviation Company air strip and all of the original Buon Le "A" — had long since been replaced by new, multiple housing units or high-rise office buildings. I didn't bother to look for those.) Emperor Bao Dai's summer palace remained (used now for public events and private affairs like weddings) but I'd felt nothing looking at it. Was it his saying, at my request, the numbers 1–10 in Rhade that I used to know by heart doing perimeter checks at the Special Forces camp in An Lac? Maybe it was simply that, on some level I'd designated Y Sam as my Montagnard "contact" and into his persona I conflated Y Rulick, H Nhe, H Yak and all the others at the hospital, and all my Montagnard patients I'd tried to help, and all the others who'd never made it to the clinic or to my sick calls, and, of course, my hospital and dispensary and aid-station colleagues, and the strikers and Truong San — just kids, really — teenagers, who had my back from time to time.

Another exception was in the Rhade longhouse, which wasn't in a Montagnard village but in a suburban neighborhood of Buon Ma Thuot, which used to be rural. After the ceremonial music, dance, and drinking, a prepared-for-tourists program, when we probed for mutual friends we discovered one, Mike Benge, my USAID representative friend. They'd known him personally, as had I. We talked about Mike — anecdotes about a Rhade girl he was sweet on, his capture by the V.C. and his years in captivity, and, on his liberation, his returning to continue to work on behalf of these people.

What was the novelty about Vietnam? First, there was the mix of the oriental and the French in architecture, and the oriental and the West in dress. Then, the near total retreat of everyone into the bosom of their families for TET, shutting down the businesses and quieting down the traffic. There was so much of unfamiliar beauty and awesome antiquity in the ancient capital city, Hue, which was doubly novel inasmuch as, unlike other Communist regimes, this one made no attempt to eradicate its non–Communist past. Instead, it celebrated it, even its French-colonial past. The places I had known were now all strangers to me. Take Buon Ho. It wasn't just that the main streets of Buon Ho were paved or that one street had two-lane traffic on each side of a tree-lined center strip. It had traffic lights, a rarity even in big cities like Hanoi. And there wasn't just one church in Buon Ho; there were four plus a cathedral!

Diane and I were the novelty in Buon Ma Thuot. The Central Highlands weren't exactly on anyone's tourist must-visit list so tourists, especially American, were almost a source of delight, maybe pride. I learned that because the Central Highlands with its Montagnards had continued, after the war, to be a source of dissent, foreigners had long been prohibited from traveling there. Tourism in BMT was a recent phenomenon; businessmen, however, were already common. Dar Lac (now Dak Lak) had become, in fact, the world's second largest coffee bean exporter after Columbia.

The architecture of the ethnic Vietnamese traditional dwelling hadn't changed over the years. Neither had the Rhade longhouse. What was novel was seeing them linked into single homes in Buon Ma Thuot's suburbs, where there had once been rural villages. Alongside the longhouses I saw no elephants as I had years before. Underneath and alongside them, instead of pigs and water buffalo, there were Italian motor scooters. These interesting hybrid homes on paved streets, with their electricity, seemed everywhere. There was clearly a Montagnard middle class. Some said they were still receiving preferential treatment to help integrate them (along with all ethnic minorities) as mainstream Vietnamese. Others seemed sure it was the government's way of

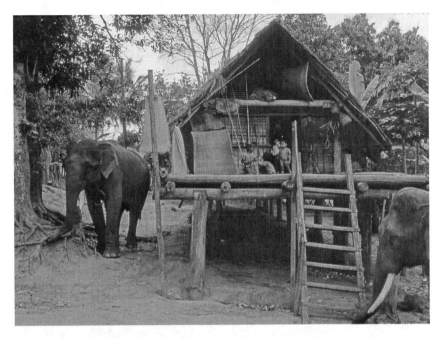

Rhade longhouse, Ban Me Thuot, 1966.

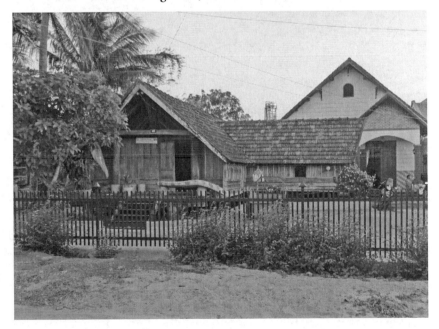

Rhade hybrid longhouse, Buon Ma Thuot, 2013 (note flag of Vietnam at the longhouse entrance).

keeping them pacified. Ought I mourn the transformation of the traditional Montagnard ways into tourist attractions? Sam told us that some of that new wealth was sent in from expatriate Montagnards who'd worked for and fought with the Americans, and had become refugees in 1975 and been accepted into America, and now were resettled in American communities like the one in Greensboro, North Carolina. There is a law school now and medical school, too, in Buon Ma Thuot. The men of the Jarai tribe were going in for medicine, I was told; the Rhade, more for teaching. Ought I feel assured? Or should I view this as akin to Chinese "integrating" Tibet because, since 2006, the Montagnards have no longer been the majority population in the Central Highlands? The ethnic Vietnamese who've relocated there now are the major-ity. With these demographic changes, I learned, deforestation and confinement with abuse by exploiters and poachers have rendered the native elephants of the highlands close to an endangered species. (I could go on.)

Novel, too, was having candid conversations with our English-speaking guides who were children, grandchildren, or nephews and nieces, of South Vietnamese soldiers and airmen, Vietcong conscripts and volunteers, North Vietnamese regular army soldiers during the Vietnam War, and Chinese-Viet-namese merchants. Novel, too, was our noticing, throughout Vietnam, no beggars, homeless, or street-people and the predominance of young people who appeared happy and smiled easily. (If there were elders, it would seem that, in the main, they kept to themselves at home. In any case, elders, we were told, didn't speak much of the old days.) Was all of this representative? Or was what we saw "managed"?

Before leaving Buon Ma Thuot we bought locally grown coffee beans to bring back to Hoan and Sa. It had been several years since our last reunion, when their second son, Andrew, and Stephanie got married.

I felt relieved to see Vietnamese easily laugh at themselves. They joke, for example, that theirs is a nation of "millionaires" inasmuch as, with inflation, it takes $2 million Vietnamese dong to reach the equivalent of $100 U.S.

We encountered no animosity towards Americans. On the contrary, Viet-namese are taught English in their public schools, not Russian or Chinese. (France still maintains private French language schools.) We were greeted everywhere with "Hello," as if anyone wealthy enough to visit Vietnam from abroad was sure to recognize that word. This, even though, in their texts and public buildings and museums, the war is presented as the "American War." Maybe, despite the absence in their texts and historical museums, of any reference to Vietnamese killing Vietnamese — that a calamitous civil war had preceded American troops — the people knew anyway. In any event I found it ironic that Communist Vietnam today looks to America to brace it against the crushing economic influence of China. (As I write this

Chuck Hagel, America's new defense secretary, is in Vietnam specifically to help build a growing military partnership between America and Vietnam.) In their eyes we appear to be that crucial to their future, and it makes me sick thinking about the 58,000 American dead over a foreign policy that became so hobbled by a language of "crusade" and images of "falling dominoes." Communist or not, Vietnam, it appears in hindsight, would have eventually and inevitably reached out to America as a friend.

In his early years as a refugee in America and then as an American, Hoan kept Diane and me current (from his reading, personal sources, and trips back to Vietnam when his parents were ailing) on conditions in Communist Vietnam. From him I was, from the beginning, appraised of the cruel and abusive treatment of all who had supported the South Vietnamese government or had worked with Americans. People were sent away for years of "re-education"— sometimes just isolation from the mainstream population so as not to contaminate them with their views, sensibilities, and memories — sometimes worse. Hoan's brother, Dinh (MILPHAP's fourth interpreter), who subsequently became a teacher, was hounded mercilessly by the Communists until he took his life. Some, of course, were sent away never to be seen or heard from again.

In the 1980s, I was told, when the man chosen to be the top figure of the Communist Party was chosen from the South, not the North, the issue of economy finally overrode issues of ideology. It was on his initiative, I learned, that what had been punitive policies regarding expatriate Vietnamese were replaced by policies favoring investment by them, encouraging them to return, even to buy property according to a "private property" designation, more like a long-term lease. (Some do, I'm told, but most don't.) The distrust of the Communists is steadfast because the government has, too many times, arbitrarily changed the rules and taken things away. Memories of entrepreneurs who'd been impoverished and disgraced by everything being taken away — "you must have made your money stealing from the People" was the mantra into the late 1970s — don't evaporate with fragile promises.

I'm sure there is envy and admiration, not just hunger for the U.S. dollar. I say this because I've been told that the Vietnamese are quick to spot an expatriate returning to visit. Their demeanor alone the way they carry themselves, gives them away. In fact, locals have even been known to try to affect these features so as to pass themselves off as returning Vietnamese Americans to hit on local girls.

In the lobby of the Renaissance Riverside Hotel in Saigon, and per plans made and confirmed by e-mail, I connected with Nguyen Chinh, Stan's interpreter. We recognized one another immediately. This was the third time I felt the connection I'd unconsciously hoped for, a reuniting with someone who was there and who knew and remembered me. How else am I to understand why grasping Chinh's hand felt the way one delightfully grasps the hand of an old and dear friend? Unfortunately, we were not able to take a cab to his house for dinner as planned, so I wasn't able to reunite with his wife who, back in 1966–67, was Co Gaiu, a head nurse at the province hospital.[1] Chinh and Diane and I had dinner at the hotel and spoke long and frankly. He, too, is a writer.

Debriefing, Family Time and One Intense Reunion

The next morning we left Vietnam for Hong Kong, a change of planes there, and then the U.S. We'd set aside a weekend in Los Angeles for a debriefing and family time with Hoan and Sa, retirees now like Diane and me, and dinners for us all at the homes our two Vietnamese nephews and their families, with Lawrence and Lien (and their son and daughter, Dylan and Delilah), and with Andrew and Stephanie. There the conversation was principally about family news and plans. In our conversations about Vietnam it became obvious that Communist Vietnam has serious catching up to do if it is to be competitive with its neighbors, avoid disillusionment of its young people who now see the unequal distribution of wealth quite clearly and want a better future for their children, and all while not being out-maneuvered by Chinese investors whose interests might prove more imperial than not.

Hoan and Sa, with Diane and me, had a luncheon with Dr. Niem where I met for the first time Katherine Vo, his granddaughter, who so innocently and effectively contributed to my revisiting my Vietnam War experience (which, in turn, led to this book). Our last get-together with Dr. Niem had been in 1992 when we'd flown in for Lawrence's wedding. At that reunion, (which included Don Horsburgh), Doctor Niem told us about the 1968 TET Offensive, his escape in 1975, and how he had come with his family to America and ended up, at the age of 50, training to be an American psychiatrist (like me).

How do I begin to explain the emotion I felt at this, our second meeting? Dr. Niem was well into his 80s and was unlikely to return to Vietnam or write his memoirs, even as part of him whispered he should. I found he carried himself with the same dignity — wearing his signature suit with sweater — as he had when he had the world on his shoulders. Nothing had changed except he moved more slowly. So, why was my contact with him colored, not with delight as with Chinh, but with alternating shades of sorrow? Was it because his sorrow somehow resonated with a sorrow of my own? But the two aren't comparable. The worlds he lost and the suffering he endured and the burden he had borne were of another order entirely than my temporary sojourn in his old world many years ago. Or was it from my guilt for the grief I visited upon him when I tried so earnestly to "hurry the East" so many years before?

Or was it because I needed a hero for that painful story that I'd come to absorb revisiting Vietnam and, in Doctor Niem, found a gentleman who had been managing those "elephants in the room" since his youth, since even before the Japanese occupation of the 1940s? And he did so holding to his dignity and honor, never "howling" or running away as I did. How could I not see his story as noble and heroic? But he will not be the story-teller of his story, and I find that sad. While, in e-mails, a part of me earnestly tried to help him begin his memoir, a part of me resisted, held back out of respect for that limited peace of mind he found, here in America, and, in spite of everything, has managed to hold on to. Did we all not see, as he was simply sharing an anecdote of witnessing injured and wounded civilians, including children, during the Communist offensive, how tears came so unexpectedly and uninvited, to silence that narrative? Enough of pain.

Doctor Niem gave me a signed copy of the book whose preparation he oversaw as president of the Overseas Imperial Family Council of Vietnam, 1995, *The House of Nguyen Phuoc: A Concise Genealogy*, his link to his country's royal past and his own, a legacy now and hard evidence of his determination and dedication, his fidelity to Vietnam's history, to family, and to the emperor. Presenting me with this book and with a personal note ,"To my old friend," it was as if he felt moved, as I did, by our connection and wanted to affirm it. It was as if he wanted to share something important and personal, as if I represented to him a kind of link in a chain. Something we're likely never to fully figure out. Maybe he was passing on to me this book of words, book of names, that told who he was and who he came from, his roots, for additional safe-keeping. In any event, our actions spoke for feelings that really had no proper words — I can't name them, maybe he can — because they weren't even invited to this luncheon in the first place. They just showed up and took me by surprise. Maybe him, too. Why else did we, in parting, shake hands with all our four hands? I'd never done that before.

The War and the MILPHAP Mission: Final Musings

America lost that war — losing a war had never happened to us. Vietnam was now united into one entity without suffering actively warring factions, and that had never happened either, at least not for a long time (and when it did, it was only for brief periods, anyway).

While Asians had, in the past, emigrated to America in large numbers, this time (the 1970s) they were not only coming in unprecedented numbers, they were welcomed and embraced, not resented, restricted, or excluded as they'd been that previous wave more than a century before. This, too, was a first for America.

Caregiving as counter insurgency, the mission of MILPHAP, was also something of a first. It wasn't GIs handing out gum or candy to hungry children, a familiar image from World War II. It wasn't "tail-gate medicine," either, something that popped up in the early 1960s and was promptly discredited. MILPHAP was a formal, full-time program, coordinated with an allied government, and it looked good on paper. But it was probably too little, too late. It also didn't work as designed for us — it couldn't — and the flash points between us and our allies were its signature symptoms. Now, as its memory seems to be disappearing into the ether, there has emerged a suggestion the program may even have done more harm than good.[2]

Communist Russia, the enemy of my childhood, collapsed, but that wasn't as much a victory of our system over theirs as it was about our system outlasting theirs, not unlike our loss in Vietnam where the will of Communist North Vietnam simply outlasted ours. It would seem you don't "win" these days. You just outlast the other guy.

MILPHAP, the humanitarian mission, was unabashedly political. It was up front and transparent, but I never personally felt a chill or sense of contamination of our humanitarian effort because of its political objective. The threat to kidnap MILPHAP doctors can not be compared with the 2012 murder of aid workers in Pakistan vaccinating against polio. The threat to kidnap a MILPHAP doctor wasn't in retaliation for any harm to their side (like our killing Bin Laden). It was simply an effort to bring that doctor to their facilities to care for their soldiers.

Postscript

A Comforting Sadness

I was credited with making mobile trips. When you think about it, wasn't I just running away from something when I set out on those trips, running away from that "double bind" I'd found myself in? It's as if a person's apparent rising to an occasion, setting himself a worthy deed to perform, a steep mountain to climb (my mobile trips into the districts) sometimes turns out to be more about accidentally running up against that "mountain" when you weren't even looking or paying attention or, in my case, were running *from* something else. Maybe, sometimes, we set out to conquer that mountain, not because of confidence in ourselves or daring in the face of challenge, but because there is an alternative that is worse. There's something on our heels, or coming from inside us, and we flee. I prefer the words "flee" and "flight" because the latter connotes a soaring with expansive exuberance, not just fear, retreat, and the need to run for cover that just happens to be in the direction of a particularly big mountain (or a dirt road into a Vietcong-infested district).

I suspect that's why the GIs at the Bungalow felt awkward about the USO performers, or their families and boosters back home, praising their "putting their lives on the line." I can imagine such statements leaving them feeling, not lauded, but unconnected, bogus, even used. I wonder if this isn't sometimes the case for soldiers awarded medals for their service when, deep down, they know they were just doing their job. (Or, in my case, not even doing their job right.)

My final, and sadly comforting, observation. This American's story is an American story. But when I step back I can see in it anyone's story, meaning it's just another Everyone's Story. We're all cut from the same cloth, part of one family. Didn't we (and don't we still) fight and even kill one another, just like members of families the world over? And then, of course, make up?

Appendix I

"Vietnamese Refugee Couple Coming to City," by Kirk Scharfenberg, printed in the *Berkshire Eagle*, Saturday, June 7, 1975.

A young Vietnamese couple, refugees from the war in their homeland, are scheduled to arrive in Pittsfield Monday to begin settling in to a new life in the Berkshires.

The couple, Nguyen Dang Hoan, 29, and his wife Tran Thi Kim Sa, 25, will reside with Dr. Lawrence H. and Diane Climo at their home at 546 South St. For 12 months in 1966 and 1967 Hoan (pronounced "Juan") served as an interpreter and medical assistant to Dr. Climo in a medical unit in Vietnam's Northern Highlands.

A week ago, Dr. Climo was informed by the American Red Cross that Hoan and his wife were at the refugee center at Ft. Chaffee, Ark. They made contact by telephone and the Climos readily agreed to act as the American sponsors for Hoan and his wife.

They are scheduled to meet at the airport in Albany on Monday. "We are very eager to get together," Dr. Climo, a psychiatrist at the Austen Riggs Center in Stockbridge, said yesterday.

Top Priority

"Helping them make the adjustment to the Pittsfield setting is our top priority," Dr. Climo. "Finding them employment is next."

For Hoan, a high school graduate, this is the third trip to the United States. He served as a pilot in South Vietnam's Air Force and was here in 1969 and again in 1971 for training at U.S. Air Force bases in Texas and Louisiana. His wife has not been here previously, but served as an information clerk in the U.S. Consulate General's Office in Nha Trang and types in English.

Because of Hoan's training with aircraft — he flew C-47s in the war — Dr. Climo believes he is best suited to some kind of work with machinery.

"They want very much to make a start and be on their own," Dr. Climo said, "and they want to do any work."

Dr. Climo said he did not yet know the specifics of the couples flight from Vietnam. Nor did he know how long they have been in the United States.

Motivation

But their motivation for leaving Vietnam is clearly spelled out in a handwritten letter sent to Dr. Climo by Hoan this week:

"We have learned that it's hard to avoid the Communists' punishment when we have many relations to which the Communists pay attention. So before deciding our departure to the United States in order to survive, we know that we will have many adjustments to do, many things must be hardships but we accept them as we must."

Dr. Climo and Hoan worked together in what was called the "Military Provincial Hospital Assistance Program" which was operated under the direction of South Vietnam's ministry of health. They worked primarily in a hospital in Ban Me Thuot, capital of the province of Dar Lac in the Northern Highlands but also made trips to dispensaries in the districts and aid stations in nearby villages and hamlets.

Their patients were exclusively civilians and Dr. Climo can recall treating two persons suffering from direct war injuries. Dr. Climo said the diseases treated included cholera, plague, smallpox, rabies, snake bites, typhoid fever, leprosy and a variety of skin infections. Many of the patients, he said, were Montagnards.

Was "Liaison"

Dr. Climo described Hoan, who was employed by the U.S. Agency for International Development, as his "liaison" with the Vietnamese. In addition to serving as interpreter, Hoan advised Dr. Climo as to "what was customary, what was respectful" in dealing with the Vietnamese.

Until the past week, the two men had not communicated since Dr. Climo left Vietnam many years ago. But, Dr. Climo said, he though of Hoan often. ("He figured as the main person of my year in Vietnam.") and considered him "a dear friend, a close personal friend."

Yet, Dr. Climo said, their relationship remained somewhat formal due to his rank as a captain in the U.S. Army and his stature as a doctor. "We weren't buddies or pals in the American sense," Dr. Climo said.

Dr. Climo has never met Hoan's wife. And Diane Climo, a member of the Pittsfield Parks and Recreation Commission and immediate past president of the Central Berkshire League of Women Voters, has never met Hoan or his wife.

Fortunately, Dr. Climo said, their home has two empty rooms and a bath on the third floor that can be utilized by the Vietnamese couple and that will give them privacy from the Climos and their two young daughters (the Climos are expecting a third child in July).

Dr. Climo said his first reaction on hearing from the Red Cross was relief that Hoan was safe and his second was excitement at the opportunity to renew their friendship.

For Hoan and his wife, the Climos clearly offer the hope of a new future. "I hope the procedures will be completed shortly," Hoan wrote Dr. Climo this week, "so we can leave the holding camp and start a new life."

Appendix II

"A telegram opened the door in escaping from Vietnam," by Kirk Scharpenberg, printed in the *Berkshire Eagle*, Saturday, June 1975.

At about 4 o'clock on the morning of March 29 — just hours after the Viet Cong had ceased their nightly mortar attack, 29 year old South Vietnamese Air Force Lt. Nguyen Dang Hoan, without orders and without a radio, piloted a C-7 cargo plane down the runway of the airfield in Danang and headed for Saigon.

It was the first step in a harrowing one month ordeal, an often terrifying and seemingly hopeless venture that would start Hoan and his 25 year-old wife on an odyssey from Vietnam , where they feared imprisonment and even death to Guam, Fort Chaffee, Ark and, finally, to Pittsfield.

They Were Lucky

During much of the time Hoan and his wife, Tran Thi Kim Sa were separated, neither knowing whether the other had survived the chaos that seized South Vietnam as the Viet Cong swept through the country. In the end, they agree, only good fortune accounts for the successful flight to the United States.

Hoan (pronounced "Juan") and Sa (pronounced "Shah") recounted the details of their flight the other day over a dinner of fried rice and chicken and a chicken and peas casserole at the home of Dr. Lawrence and Diane Climo at 546 South St. Hoan served as interpreter for Dr. Climo in Vietnam in 1966 and 1967 and the Climos are acting as the Hoans' sponsors here.

Hoan said he, along with 23 other members of the South Vietnamese Air Force, decided to flee Danang in the cargo plane when it became clear that the air base was about to fall to the Viet Cong. Senior officers, he said, had already fled leaving behind no evacuation plans.

The hurried early morning flight prevented Hoan from contacting his wife who was in Nha Trang where she had worked for seven years for the American Consulate General's office, a connection with the United States that was to be the Hoans' eventually passport to safety.

When Hoan arrived at the Saigon air field — he was guided in by lights from the ground — he and the others on the plane were assigned to another Air Force unit. Two days later he learned that the consulate office in Nha Trang had been closed and the staff was being flown to Saigon.

Missed the Flight

Hoan went to the airport to meet Sa, but she had missed the flight and did not arrive. Hoan then journeyed to Vung Tau, a port city east of Saigon to await Sa's arrival by ship. For three days he waited but she did not arrive. "My skin," Hoan said, "was like the skin of a chicken."

Meanwhile, to the north in Nha Trang Sa, a sister, and her father, who was a police official in Nha Trang, had taken refuge in a Catholic church, seeking safety from the Viet Cong, fleeing South Vietnamese soldiers and former prisoners who had escaped from the jails in the area and were robbing and assaulting civilians.

After she had spent three days in the church, a ship was spotted off the coast of Nha Trang. Thousands of refugees inside the city rushed to the nearby deep-water port and attempted to jump on a large barge tied to a dock there. Two thousand, Sa estimated, made it. Scores failed and drowned.

The barge was towed out to the ship where its passengers joined 3,000 persons already aboard for a week-long trip to Phuquoc, an island south of Saigon where the South Vietnamese government had established a camp for refugees from the northern part of the country.

Sa was in a massive camp there for a week. Civilians were not permitted to leave because the government was afraid an influx of refugees into Saigon would set off a panic there. Sa and Hoan had still no contact.

Telegram Did It

Finally, Sa prepared a telegram addressed to a brother in Saigon and with it walked six miles to the periphery of the camp, passing by five police checkpoints by posing as a vendor. At the gate she was able to convince a soldier to send the telegram.

Her family received the message and brought it to the consulate general's office in Saigon which arranged for a plane to fly to Phuquoc to pick up employees of American agencies camped there. Sa was flown to Saigon where she was finally reunited with her husband.

While, as a rule, South Vietnamese military men were not permitted to join the wave of refugees fleeing Vietnam, Hoan, because of his wife's position with the United States government, was permitted to join her and 10 members of her family on a flight to Guam on April 27.

About ten days later, Hoan and Sa were flown to Fort Chaffee. About three weeks ago they established contact with the Climos and less than two weeks ago they arrived in Pittsfield. The 10 members of Sa's family who accompanied them on the flight to Guam are now at Camp Pendleton studying English and hoping that American sponsors can be arranged for them.

Hoan is now looking for work here and has had several job interviews. Eventually, he said, he would like to get a pilot's license, though he realizes that will take time and money. He is patient. "Since we arrive in Guam," he said, "we feel very safe and very happy."

Appendix III

On April 7, 1968, two months after the 1968 TET Offensive, a medical officer of the 734th Medical Detachment, MILPHAP, wrote me in reply to my inquiry.

Dear Dr. Climo, I'm sorry about the delay answering your letter. Things have been very busy. I'm the only military doctor (MILPHAP or MACV Team 33) here now and have been out of town a couple of times besides. Don (Horsburgh) went back to the states at the end of January, about 2 months early.

Dr. Niem is regional medical chief and hospital chief. The military surgeon is province medicine chief. Dr. Niem is in Saigon at the moment and will probably be appointed to a political medicine position there.

The interpreter Nguyen Dang Hoan was drafted. I'll try to get his current address. Ba Nam is still working in OPD. (I think she must be the same Co Nam you asked about.) Y Blo is in OPD. Mr. Tom has been in the clinic but is now on the public health staff.

The program is changing. We are no longer a Provincial Hospital Assistance Program but a Public Health Assistance Program. People are being assigned to specific divisions such as malaria program, health education, etc. to get these programs functioning as they were designed to do. We do have members assigned at Phuc An, Buon Ho, and Lac Thien, working in the subsector medical programs. We are employing fewer people in the hospital and expecting the Vietnamese to do more.

Ban Me Thuot was considered about 20 percent destroyed. This included all the Vietnamese part of Buon Ali A (sic) and much of the Rhade part, almost all of the city behind Sector and on the street between Sector and the province chief's house, several blocks downtown and scattered blocks in other sections of town. The entire mission house complex was destroyed. Much of the town now has sand bags and bunkers. It is much more grim than before.

We had been receiving regular mortar attacks in the city There have been many civilian casualties. This appears to be decreasing now.

The new hospital buildings are progressing rapidly. You wouldn't recognize the hospital grounds now. Construction includes outpatient facility, surgical ward, pediatric ward, enlarged operating suite, water tower, electric generator, as well as remodeling of the old surgical ward, warehouse, and kitchen.

If you are interested in any other progress here, drop a line from time to time.

Appendix IV

John Guingrich, personal communication

I was drafted along with all my other classmates from Grade School, High School, and Sunday School — all young men from the fields and factories of rural and small town America. And because a good many of us were from the same (Anabaptist) background and faith — we were inducted as Conscientious Objectors to be trained as Combat Medics in Non-Combatant military roles. It was never our intent to dodge service. We were thankful to live in a country under a benevolent government that allowed us to serve our country. The men I served with — I believe we all shared a similar ideal of why we were there and what was expected of us. And after being there for a year among the people of South Vietnam I would have to say it would have been easy to either have stayed on or gone back there to live among those people. When

I finally did arrive home I was thunder-struck by the massive anti-war rioting I encountered on the Capitol Grounds in Washington DC.

During my subsequent career as a facility engineer at Caterpillar Inc. I was privileged to have a good friend who I worked with and who had grown up in Saigon. We would take lunch about the same time every day and getting to know him and work with him over the years was an added bonus and unexpected blessing that certainly went a long way toward erasing any bad memories I may have hidden in my experience. His struggle to reach American shores as a boat person were incredible. In his own close knit family there were officers and pilots who fought on both sides of the conflict — In all these years since — the thing I still cannot reconcile is what on earth was this argument about anyway.

My oldest sister, Carol and her husband after having raised a large family of their own, sponsored and adopted a beautiful Vietnamese teenager whose struggle for survival as a boat person is a humbling tribute to the grace and courage that has enriched our lives through the many Vietnamese refugees that came to our shores. The sacrifices laid down in blood by the soldiers who simply did their duty as they saw it — and who then came back home to pick up their lives in a country that is today more divided as a nation than we have ever been in our collective memory — well for me — all I have to do is look at a Vietnamese refugee of that struggle, and quietly reflect that it was worthwhile. I will always have that to take with me.

Chapter Notes

Chapter 1

1. According to Bernard Fall, "Cochin" was how Marco Polo mispronounced the Chinese "Giao-chi," their name for this place, and the word "China" was added for geographic clarification. "Cochinchina" was for several centuries the name under which Viet-Nam was best known in the West (Bernard B. Hall, *The Two Viet-Nams: A Political and Military Analysis* [New York: Frederick A. Praeger, 1966], 19).

2. Hall, *Two Viet-Nams*, 25.

3. Robert Shaplen, *The Lost Revolution: The U.S. in Vietnam*, 1946–1966 (New York: Harper and Row, 1966), 78.

4. "None of the participants actually signed but simply 'took note,' individually" (Shaplen, *Lost Revolution*, 96).

5. Shaplen, *Lost Revolution*, 132.

6. Ahmad Eqbal, "The Policy of the Government of the Republic of (South) [*sic*] Vietnam with Regard to Former Resistance Members," in Marvin E. Gettleman, ed., *Vietnam: History, Documents, and Opinions on a Major World Crisis* (Greenwich: Fawcett, 1965), 361.

7. Gettleman, *Vietnam: History, Documents, and Opinions on a Major World Crisis*, 191–192.

8. The Rhade were the first to participate. Since 1961 they'd already been part of a highly successful program whereby the U.S. Mission provided weapons and training and the Rhade provided a village self-defense program. By 1962, 40 villages were thus secured. However, when the Americans turned command over to Vietnamese Special Forces officers, the Rhade soldiers would, in time, quit the program because their Vietnamese officers would repeat old habits of disdain, disrespect, and abuse.

9. Philippe Devillers, "Ngo Dinh Diem and the Struggle for Reunification in Vietnam," in Gettleman, ed., *Vietnam*, 233.

10. David Halberstam, "The Buddhist Crisis in Vietnam: A Pulitzer Prize-Winning Report," in Gettleman, ed., *Vietnam*, 264.

11. Congressional Record, "'Vietnam and the National Interest,' by Hans J. Morgenthau, the selection is from 'We Are Deluding Ourselves in Vietnam,' *The New York Times Magazine* (April 18, 1965), by permission," cited in Gettleman, ed., *Vietnam*, 376.

12. Adam Clymer, "Barry Goldwater, Conservative and Individualist, Dies at 89," May 1998, http://www.nytimes.com/books/01/04/01/specials/goldwater-obit.html.

13. Congressional Record, "'Dissent in the Senate (1963-1965),' September 6, 1963. Selections from the *Congressional Record*. (These selections have appeared in the Marzani and Munsell pamphlet, the *Conscience of the Senate* (New York, 1965), which must be used with great care because some speeches are quoted there out of context to give the appearance of greater dissent than actually exists. In each case I have checked the context of the speech.—ed.)," cited in Gettleman, ed., *Vietnam*, 387.

Chapter 3

1. Salinas, California was not a "home town" in the fullest sense. Rodriguez writes: "I dropped out of high-school cause my father needed help with ten kids including me. Was a migrant worker for a while, moved to San Joaquin Valley near Fresno, California. Lived in a labor camp and paid room and board. Moved to Salinas and got a job. Saved enough to bring my parents to California. My dad reminded me of Grapes of Wrath when he showed up in a car with my Mom and eight kids" (personal communication).

2. Lightweight, prefabricated structures of corrugated galvanized steel with a semicircular cross-section that could be shipped anywhere and assembled without skilled labor; the two ends were covered with plywood that had doors and windows cut out. Used during World War II for housing, offices, barracks, latrines.

Chapter 5

1. In the 1960s villages formed local militias for protection. They were called Civil Guard and Self-Defense Corps. In 1964 they were integrated into ARVN, the Republic of Vietnam Army, and renamed Popular Forces and Regional Forces (RF-PFs).

2. The 155th, which had an air field and lots of helicopters outside town, patrolled the area and made medical evacuations when they weren't moving RVN troops, stationed nearby, into the field.

3. For perspective on this difference, note that in the spring off 1956 MAAG had taken over responsibility for reorganizing and retraining the Vietnamese Army and, under their direction, this force was rebuilt primarily along conventional lines, meaning it was meant to withstand a large scale attack from the north. They were prepped for a defensive holding operation until South East Asia Treaty Organization (SEATO) troops could come to their aid. The Republic of Vietnam army, in other words, was trained along conventional lines, not in guerrilla tactics. RVN forces were regularly defeated. When Ranger-type forces were subsequently trained, modeled on the early success of village Self-Defense Corps, it seemed too late (Shaplen, *Lost Revolution*, 138–39).

4. Six national flags have flown over Texas since the first European exploration of the region by Cortez in 1519. These are Texas under Spain (1919–1685; 1690–1821), Texas under France (1685–1690), Texas under Mexico (1821–1836), Texas as a Republic (1836–1845), Texas in the Confederacy (1861–1865), and Texas in the U.S. (1845–1861; 1865–present).

Chapter 6

1. A naturally occurring aromatic compound with slight anesthetic and antimicrobial actions, taken orally or applied to skin as a folk remedy for treating fatigue; toxic in high doses.

2. Michael D. Benge, "The History of the Involvement of the Montagnards of the Central Highlands in the Vietnam War," December 2010, Folder 01, Box 01, Michael D. Benge Collection, The Vietnam Center and Archive, Texas Tech University, accessed 24 March 2013, <http://www.vietnam.ttu.edu/virtualarchive/items.php?item=24090101001>.

3. From the Benge online article: "Traditionally, the average Vietnamese viewed the highlands as an abode of evil malevolent spirits; as a place where 'poisoned water' (nuóc độc) flowed in the streams; a region of forested mountains teeming with Moi (savages — the term Vietnamese used when referring to Montagnards) with poison-tipped arrows; and a region populated with huge ferocious tigers and other jungle beasts. Few Vietnamese ventured into the Central Highlands during French colonization; it was an exception rather than the rule, however, that a few Vietnamese traders braved the Highlands, and the French had brought in a few others in administrative positions. After the French established rubber, coffee and tea plantations in the Highlands, Vietnamese elite began to envy the French and greedily covet the Highlands for its rich

potential in resources of 'fertile' soils, minerals, hardwoods, cinnamon and other forest products. After the disastrous defeats of the French in the Central Highlands and at Dien Bien Phu, the politicians and generals, both in the North and the South, began to see that strategically, whoever controls the highlands would eventually control Vietnam.

Chapter 12

1. For a more details and follow-up of this young soldier see Appendix V.

2. "His name is Y Suah Buon Krong. (I'm not sure of the spelling; there are all sorts of diacritical marks that I don't remember.) He was very good to work with. We had all the equipment to do WBC differential counts except for the mechanical tabulator, basically a button for each kind of WBC and a bell that rang when you'd counted to 100. Cost over $100. Y Suah showed me how to fold a box out of paper for each type of WBC and then start with 100 beans and put them in the appropriate boxes until I ran out. Low-tech but a lot cheaper and just as efficient. I can still count to 100 in Vietnamese. I also remember one day early in our rotation he pitched sideways off his chair. I didn't know if he'd been shot or had a heart attack or what. Turns out he was epileptic. He was all right. He gifted me a bottle of rice wine and I think I drank it in my room. I don't remember if I shared it or not. I hope I did" (Daniel Melberg, personal communication).

Chapter 13

1. The fourth chapter in Sam Korsmoe's book of narratives, *Saigon Stories*, tells the stories of both Chinh and Giao and includes many of the details shared at our reunion.

2. Robert J. Wilensky, M.D., a battalion medical officer in Vietnam 1967–68 who went on to receive a Ph.D. in history from American University in 2000 and authored the 2004 book *Military Medicine to Win Hearts and Minds*, posits that programs like MILPHAP may have actually done more harm than good. How? By making obvious the inability of the South Vietnamese government to provide basic health care to its people, and the difference between the caring demonstrated by American caregivers compared to their own countrymen.

Bibliography

Baker, Major Jay B. "Military Diplomacy in Full-Spectrum Operations." *Military Review*, September–October 2007, 67–73.

Benge, Michael Dennis. "Benge, Michael Dennis." www.pownetwork.org/blos/b/b600. htm. Accessed March 24, 2013.

_____. "The History of the Involvement of the Montagnards of the Central Highlands in the Vietnam War." In *"The Fall of Saigon," SACEI Forum #8*, March 2011. Outskirts Press.com.

_____. "The History of the Involvement of the Montagnards of the Central Highlands in the Vietnam War." December 2010. Folder 01, Box 01, Michael D. Benge Collection, The Vietnam Center and Archive, Texas Tech University. http://www.vietnam.ttu. edu/virtualarchive/items.php?item=24090101001. Accessed March 24, 2013.

Bowman, John S., ed. *The Vietnam War: An Almanac*. New York: World Almanac, 1985.

Burns, Charles. *Our War: Buon Ho, Vietnam 1966–67*. Self-published, 2008.

Climo, Lawrence H. "Doctor to the Montagnards." *Vietnam*, December 1999, 48–52.

_____. "Unorthodox Practice: An American Doctor in Vietnam." *Vietnam*, April 2003, 26–32.

Fall, Bernard B. *Street Without Joy: From the Indochina War to the War in Vietnam*. Harrisburg: Stackpole, 1964

_____. *The Two Viet-Nams: A Political and Military Analysis*. New York: Frederick A. Praeger, 1966.

Gettleman, Marvin E., ed. *Vietnam: History, Documents, and Opinions on a Major World Crisis*. Greenwich: Fawcett, 1965.

Giap, General Vo Nguyen. *People's War People's Army: The Viet Cong Insurrection Manual for Underdeveloped Countries*. New York: Frederick A. Prager, 1965.

Kirkland, Faris R. "Cultural Dynamics of Civic Action in the Central Highlands of Vietnam, 1967–68." *Armed Forces and Society: An Interdisciplinary Journal* 26.4 (June 2000): 547–60.

Korsmoe, Sam. *Saigon Stories*. Baltimore: Publish America, 2006.

Lacouture, Jean. *Vietnam: Between Two Truces*. New York: Vintage, 1966.

Laurence, John. *The Cat from Hue: A Vietnam War Story*. New York: Public Affairs, 2002.

Lifton, Robert Jan. *Home from the War: Vietnam Veterans, Neither Victims nor Executioners*. New York: Simon and Schuster, 1873.

O'Brien, Tim. *The Things They Carried*. New York: Mariner, 1990

Raskin, Marcus G., and Bernard B. Fall, eds. *The Viet-Nam Reader: Articles and Documents on American Foreign Policy and the Viet-Nam Crisis*. New York: Vintage, 1965.

Shaplen, Robert. *The Lost Revolution: The U.S. in Vietnam, 1946–66.* New York: Harper and Row, 1966.

Sochurek, Howard "American Special Forces in Action in Viet Nam: "How Coolness and Character Averted a Blood Bath When Mountain Tribesmen Rose in Revolt." *National Geographic* January 1965; 127:38–65.

Warner, Denis. *The Last Confucian.* New York: Macmillian, 1963.

Wilensky, Robert. *Military Medicine to Win Hearts and Minds: Aid to Civilians in the Vietnam War.* Texas Tech University Press, 2004.

Index

Page numbers in **_bold italics_** indicate pages with illustrations.